Test Yourself

Biological Psychology

Test Yourself... Psychology Series

Test Yourself

Biological Psychology

Dominic Upton and Penney Upton

Multiple-Choice Questions prepared by Emma L. Preece

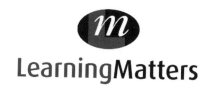

LearningMatters

First published in 2011 by Learning Matters Ltd

British Library Cataloguing in Publication Data
A CIP record for this book is available from the British Library
ISBN: 978 0 85725 649 2

This book is also available in the following e-book formats:
Adobe ebook ISBN: 978 0 85725 651 5
EPUB book ISBN: 978 0 85725 650 8
Kindle ISBN: 978 0 85725 652 2

Cover design by Toucan Design
Text design by Toucan Design
Project Management by Deer Park Productions, Tavistock
Typeset by Pantek Media, Maidstone, Kent
Printed and bound in Great Britain by MPG Books Group, Bodmin, Cornwall

Learning Matters Ltd
20 Cathedral Yard
Exeter
EX1 1HB
Tel: 01392 215560
info@learningmatters.co.uk
www.learningmatters.co.uk

Contents

Acknowledgements

The production of this series has been a rapid process with an apparent deadline at almost every turn. We are therefore grateful to colleagues both from Learning Matters (Julia Morris and Helen Fairlie) and the University of Worcester for making this process so smooth and (relatively) effortless. In particular we wish to thank our colleagues for providing many of the questions, specifically:

- Biological Psychology: Emma Preece
- Cognitive Psychology: Emma Preece
- Developmental Psychology: Charlotte Taylor
- Personality and Individual Differences: Daniel Kay
- Research Methods and Design in Psychology: Laura Scurlock-Evans
- Social Psychology: Laura Scurlock-Evans

Finally, we must, once again, thank our children (Gabriel, Rosie and Francesca) for not being as demanding as usual during the process of writing and development.

Introduction

Psychology is one of the most exciting subjects that you can study at university in the twenty-first century. A degree in psychology helps you to understand and explain thought, emotion and behaviour. You can then apply this knowledge to a range of issues in everyday life including health and well-being, performance in the workplace, education – in fact any aspect of life you can think of! However, a degree in psychology gives you much more than a set of 'facts' about mind and behaviour; it will also equip you with a wide range of skills and knowledge. Some of these, such as critical thinking and essay writing, have much in common with humanities subjects, while others such as hypothesis testing and numeracy are scientific in nature. This broad-based skill set prepares you exceptionally well for the workplace – whether or not your chosen profession is in psychology. Indeed, recent evidence suggests employers appreciate the skills and knowledge of psychology graduates. A psychology degree really can help you get ahead of the crowd. However, in order to reach this position of excellence, you need to develop your skills and knowledge fully and ensure you complete your degree to your highest ability.

This book is designed to enable you, as a psychology student, to maximise your learning potential by assessing your level of understanding and your confidence and competence in biological psychology, one of the core knowledge domains for psychology. It does this by providing you with essential practice in the types of questions you will encounter in your formal university assessments. It will also help you make sense of your results and identify your strengths and weaknesses. This book is one part of a series of books designed to assist you with learning and developing your knowledge of psychology. The series includes books on:

- Biological Psychology
- Cognitive Psychology
- Developmental Psychology
- Personality and Individual Differences
- Research Methods and Design in Psychology
- Social Psychology

In order to support your learning this book includes over 200 targeted Multiple-Choice Questions (MCQs) and Extended Multiple-Choice Questions (EMCQs) that have been carefully put together to help assess your depth of knowledge of biological psychology. The MCQs are split into two formats: the foundation level questions are about your level of understanding of the key principles and components of key areas in psychology.

Hopefully, within these questions you should recognise the correct answer from the four options. The advanced level questions require more than simple recognition – some will require recall of key information, some will require application of this information and others will require synthesis of information. At the end of each chapter you will find a set of essay questions covering each of the topics. These are typical of the kinds of question that you are likely to encounter during your studies. In each chapter, the first essay question is broken down for you using a concept map, which is intended to help you develop a detailed answer to the question. Each of the concept maps is shaded to show you how topics link together, and includes cross-references to relevant MCQs in the chapter. You should be able to see a progression in your learning from the foundation to the advanced MCQs, to the extended MCQs and finally the essay questions. The book is divided up into 10 chapters and your biological psychology module is likely to have been divided into similar topic areas. However, do not let this restrict your thinking in relation to biological psychology: these topics interact. The sample essay questions, which complement the questions provided in the chapter, will help you to make the links between different topic areas. You will find the answers to all of the MCQs and EMCQs at the end of the book. There is a separate table of answers for each chapter; use the self monitoring column in each of the tables to write down your own results, coding correct answers as NC, incorrect answers as NI and any you did not respond to as NR. You can then use the table on page 97 to analyse your results.

The aim of the book is not only to help you revise for your exams, it is also intended to help with your learning. However, it is not intended to replace lectures, seminars and tutorials, or to supersede the book chapters and journal articles signposted by your lecturers. What this book can do, however, is set you off on a sound footing for your revision and preparation for your exams. In order to help you to consolidate your learning, the book also contains tips on how to approach MCQ assessments and how you can use the material in this text to assess, *and enhance*, your knowledge base and level of understanding.

Now you know the reasons behind this book and how it will enhance your success, it is time for you to move on to the questions – let the fun begin!

Assessing your interest, competence and confidence

The aim of this book is to help you to maximise your learning potential by assessing your level of understanding, confidence and competence in core issues in psychology. So how does it do this?

Assessing someone's knowledge of a subject through MCQs might at first glance seem fairly straightforward: typically the MCQ consists of a question, one correct answer and one or more incorrect answers, sometimes called distractors. For example, in this book each question has one right answer and three distractors. The goal of an MCQ test is for you to get every question right and so show just how much knowledge you have. However, because you are given a number of answers to select from, you might be able to choose the right answer either by guessing or by a simple process of elimination – in other words by knowing what is not the right answer. For this reason it is sometimes argued that MCQs only test knowledge of facts rather than in-depth understanding of a subject. However, there is increasing evidence that MCQs can also be valuable at a much higher level of learning, if used in the right way (see, for example, Gardner-Medwin and Gahan, 2003). They can help you to develop as a self-reflective learner who is able to recognise the interest you have in a subject matter as well as your level of competence and confidence in your own knowledge.

MCQs can help you gauge your interest, competence and confidence in the following way. It has been suggested (Howell, 1982) that there are four possible states of knowledge (see Table 1). Firstly, it is possible that you do not know something and are not aware of this lack of knowledge. This describes the naive learner – think back to your first week at university when you were a 'fresher' student and had not yet begun your psychology course. Even if you had done psychology at A level, you were probably feeling a little self-conscious and uncertain in this new learning environment. During the first encounter in a new learning situation most of us feel tentative and unsure of ourselves; this is because we don't yet know what it is we don't know – although to feel this lack of certainty suggests that we know there is something we don't know, even if we don't yet know what this is! In contrast, some people appear to be confident and at ease even in new learning situations; this is not usually because they already know everything but rather because they too do not yet know what it is they do not know – but they have yet to even acknowledge that there is a gap in their knowledge. The next step on from this 'unconscious non-competence' is 'conscious non-competence'; once you started your psychology course you began to realise what the gaps were in your knowledge – you now knew what you didn't know! While this can be an uncomfortable feeling, it is important for the learning process that this acknowledgement of a gap in knowledge is made, because it is the first step in reaching the next level of learning – that of a 'conscious competent' learner. In other words you need to know what the gap in your knowledge is so that you can fill it.

Table 1 Consciousness and competence in learning

	Unconscious	Conscious
Non-competent	You don't know something and are not aware that you lack this knowledge/skill.	You don't know something and are aware that you lack this knowledge/skill.
Competent	You know something but are not aware of your knowledge/skill.	You know something and are aware of your knowledge/skill.

One of the ways this book can help you move from unconscious non-competency to conscious competency should by now be clear – it can help you identify the gaps in your knowledge. However, if used properly it can do much more; it can also help you to assess your consciousness and competence in this knowledge.

When you answer an MCQ, you will no doubt have a feeling about how confident you are about your answer: 'I know the answer to question 1 is A. Question 2 I am not so sure about. I am certain the answer is not C or D, so it must be A or B. Question 3, I haven't got a clue so I will say D – but that is a complete guess.' Sound familiar? Some questions you know the answers to, you have that knowledge and know you have it; other questions you are less confident about but think you may know which (if not all) are the distractors, while for others you know this is something you just don't know. Making use of this feeling of confidence will help you become a more reflective – and therefore effective – learner.

Perhaps by now you are wondering where we are going with this and how any of this can help you learn. 'Surely all that matters is whether or not I get the answers right? Does that show I have knowledge?' Indeed it may well do and certainly, if you are confident in your answers, then yes it does. But what if you were not sure? What if your guess of D for our fictional question 3 above was correct? What if you were able to complete all the MCQs in a test and score enough to pass – but every single answer was a guess? Do you really know and understand psychology because you have performed well – and will you be able to do the same again if you retake the test next week? Take a look back at Table 1. If you are relying on guesswork and hit upon the answer by accident you might perform well without actually understanding how you know the answer, or that you even knew it (unconscious competence), or you may not realise you don't know something (unconscious non-competence). According to this approach to using MCQs what is important is not how many answers you get right, but whether or not you acknowledge your confidence in the answer you give: it is better to get a wrong answer and acknowledge it is wrong (so as to work on filling that gap).

Therefore what we recommend you do when completing the MCQs is this: for each answer you give, think about how confident you are that it is right. You might want to rate each of your answers on the following scale:

3:    I am confident this is the right answer.

2:    I am not sure, but I think this is the right answer.

1:    I am not sure, but I think this is the wrong answer.

0:    I am confident this is the wrong answer.

Using this system of rating your confidence will help you learn for yourself both what you know and what you don't know. You will become a conscious learner through the self-directed activities contained in this book. Reflection reinforces the links between different areas of your learning and knowledge and strengthens your ability to *justify* an answer, so enabling you to perform to the best of your ability.

References

Gardner-Medwin, A. R. and Gahan, M. (2003) *Formative and Summative Confidence-Based Assessment*, Proceedings of 7th International Computer-Aided Assessment Conference, Loughborough, UK, July, pp. 147–55.

Howell, W. C. (1982) 'An overview of models, methods, and problems', in W.C. Howell and E.A. Fleishman (eds), *Human Performance and Productivity, Vol. 2: Information Processing and Decision Making*. Hillsdale, NJ: Erlbaum.

Tips for success: how to succeed in your assessments

This book, part of a comprehensive new series, will help you achieve your psychology aspirations. It is designed to assess your knowledge so that you can review your current level of performance and where you need to spend more time and effort reviewing and revising material. However, it hopes to do more than this – it aims to assist you with your learning so it not only acts as an assessor of performance but as an aid to learning. Obviously, it is not a replacement for every single text, journal article, presentation and abstract you will read and review during the course of your degree programme. Similarly, it is in no way a replacement for your lectures, seminars or additional reading – it should complement all of this material. However, it will also add something to all of this other material: learning is assisted by reviewing and assessing and this is what this text aims to do – help you learn through assessing your learning.

The focus throughout this book, as it is in all of the books in this series, is on how you should approach and consider your topics in relation to assessment and exams. Various features have been included to help you build up your skills and knowledge ready for your assessments.

This book, and the other companion volumes in this series, should help you learn through testing and assessing yourself – it should provide an indication of how advanced your thinking and understanding is. Once you have assessed your understanding you can explore what you need to learn and how. However, hopefully, quite a bit of what you read here you will already have come across and the text will act as a reminder and set your mind at rest – you do know your material.

Succeeding at MCQs

Exams based on MCQs are becoming more and more frequently used in higher education and particularly in psychology. As such you need to know the best strategy for completing such assessments and succeeding. The first thing to note is, if you know the material then the questions will present no problems – so revise and understand your notes and back this up with in-depth review of material presented in textbooks, specialist materials and journal articles. However, once you have done this you need to look at the technique for answering multiple-choice questions and here are some tips for success:

1. Time yourself. The first important thing to note when you are sitting your examination is the time available to you for completing it. If you have, for example, an hour and a half to answer 100 multiple-choice questions this means you have 54 seconds to complete each question. This means that you have to read, interpret, think about and select one answer for a multiple-choice question in under a minute. This may seem impossible, but there are several things that you can do to use your time effectively.

2. Practise. By using the examples in this book, those given out in your courses, in class tests, or on the web you can become familiar with the format and wording of multiple-choice questions similar to those used in your exam. Another way of improving your chances is to set your own multiple-choice exams – try and think of some key questions and your four optional responses (including the correct one of course!). Try and think of optional distractors that are sensible and not completely obvious. You could, of course, swap questions with your peers – getting them to set some questions for you while you set some questions for them. Not only will this help you with your practice but you will also understand the format of MCQs and the principles underlying their construction – this will help you answer the questions when it comes to the real thing.

3. The rule of totality. Look out for words like 'never' and 'always' in multiple-choice questions. It is rare in psychology for any answer to be true in relation to these words of 'totality'. As we all know, psychology is a multi-modal subject that has multiple perspectives and conflicting views and so it is very unlikely that there will always be a 'never' or an 'always'. When you see these words, focus on them and consider them carefully. A caveat is, of course, sometimes never and always will appear in a question, but be careful of these words!

4. Multiple, multiple-choice answers. Some multiple-choice answers will contain statements such as 'both A and C' or 'all of the above' or 'none of these'. Do not be distracted by these choices. Multiple-choice questions have only one correct answer and do not ask for opinion or personal bias. Quickly go through each choice independently, crossing off the answers that you know are not true. If, after eliminating the incorrect responses, you think there is more than one correct answer, group your answers and see if one of the choices matches yours. If you believe only one answer is correct, do not be distracted by multiple-choice possibilities.

5. 'First guess is best' fallacy. There is a myth among those who take (or even write) MCQs that the 'first guess is best'. This piece of folklore is misleading: research (and psychologists love research) indicates that when people change their answers on an MCQ exam, about two-thirds of the time they go from wrong to right, showing that the first guess is often not the best. So, think about it and consider your answer – is it right? Remember, your first guess is not better than a result obtained through good, hard, step-by-step, conscious thinking that enables you to select the answer that you believe to be the best.

6. The rule of threes. One of the most helpful strategies for multiple-choice questions is a three-step process:

(i)   Read the question thoroughly but quickly. Concentrate on particular words such as 'due to' and 'because' or 'as a result of' and on words of totality such as 'never' or 'always' (although see rule 3 above).

(ii)   Rather than going to the first answer you think is correct (see rule 5) eliminate the ones that you think are wrong one by one. While this may take more time, it is more likely to provide the correct answer. Furthermore, answer elimination may provide a clue to a misread answer you may have overlooked.

(iii) Reread the question, as if you were reading it for the first time. Now choose your answer from your remaining answers based on this rereading.

7. Examine carefully. Examine each of the questions carefully, particularly those that are very similar. It may be that exploring parts of the question will be useful – circle the parts that are different. It is possible that each of the alternatives will be very familiar and hence you must **understand the meaning** of each of the alternatives with respect to the context of the question. You can achieve this by studying for the test as though it will be a short-answer or essay test. Look for the level of **qualifying words**. Such words as *best, always, all, no, never, none, entirely, completely* suggest that a condition exists without exception. Items containing words that provide for some level of exception or qualification are: *often, usually, less, seldom, few, more* and *most* (and see rule 3). If you know that two or three of the options are correct, **'all of the above'** is a strong possibility.

8. Educated guesses. Never leave a question unanswered. If nothing looks familiar, pick the answer that seems most complete and contains the most information. Most of the time (if not all of the time!) the best way to answer a question is to know the answer! However, there may be times when you will not know the answer or will not really understand the question. There are three circumstances in which you should guess: when you are stuck, when you are running out of time, or both of these! Guessing strategies are always dependent on the scoring system used to mark the exam (see the section on MCQ scoring mechanisms). If the multiple-choice scoring system makes the odds of gaining points equal to the odds of having points deducted it does not pay to guess if you are unable to eliminate any of the answers. But the odds of improving your test score are in your favour if you can rule out even one of the answers. The odds in your favour increase as you rule out more answers in any one question. So, take account of the scoring mechanisms and then eliminate, move onwards and guess!

9. Revise and learn. Study carefully and learn your material. The best tip for success is always to learn the material. Use this book, use your material, use your time wisely but, most of all, use your brain!

Chapter 1
Introduction to biological psychology

This chapter provides questions relating to the biological bases of contemporary psychology. It includes topics such as schools of thought, the scope of the subject, key terms and concepts, methodological considerations and prominent milestones in research. It will test both your foundation and advanced knowledge of these topics. At the end of the chapter are several example essay questions and a sample concept map which may enable you to organise your thoughts during essay planning.

Select one answer for each question.

Foundation level questions

1. Which of the following contains an item which is not a branch of neuroscience?

    A. Neuroanatomy, computational neuroscience, molecular neuroscience.

    B. Neurochemistry, neurolinguistics, behavioural neuroscience.

    C. Neuropharmacology, neuropathology, neuroendocrinology.

    D. None of the above.

Your answer: ☐

2. Reductionism is the term applied to which of the following practices?

    A. Explaining complex phenomena in terms of simpler processes.

    B. Explaining simple phenomena in terms of complex processes.

    C. Explaining complex phenomena in terms of equally complex processes.

    D. Explaining simple phenomena in terms of equally simple processes.

Your answer: ☐

3. Attempts to gain physiological understanding by studying normal function would be advocated by which school of thought?

A. Structuralism.

B. Functionalism.

C. Dualism.

D. Behaviourism.

Your answer: ☐

4. An automatic motor response produced as a direct result of a stimulus is known as which of the following?

A. Visuomotor.

B. Unilateral neglect.

C. Reflex.

D. Generalisation.

Your answer: ☐

5. The belief that behaviour can be modified and regulated using conditioning is consistent with which school of thought?

A. Behaviourism.

B. Cognitivism.

C. Connectionism.

D. Neuropsychology.

Your answer: ☐

6. Which of the following schools of thought correspond with the belief that 'mind' is a phenomenon produced by the nervous system?

A. Dualism.

B. Monism.

C. Phenomenology.

D. Introspection.

Your answer: ☐

7. What is the evolutionary function of genetic mutation?

    A. Creating genetic consistency.

    B. Irradiating difference in a gene pool.

    C. Encouraging reproduction.

    D. Creating genetic variability.

Your answer: ☐

8. Müller (1801–58) established which of the following theories?

    A. Doctrine of specific nerve energies.

    B. Experimental ablation.

    C. Functionalism.

    D. Structuralism.

Your answer: ☐

9. Which of the following is the correct definition of blindsight?

    A. Skills displayed by individuals who are blind from birth.

    B. Ability to reach for objects in the blind field without conscious perception.

    C. Visual processing without the influence of the visual spotlight.

    D. Perception not involving any region of the brain.

Your answer: ☐

10. Which of the following can be severed in an attempt to reduce the effects of epilepsy?

    A. Brain stem.

    B. Amygdala.

    C. Corpus callosum.

    D. Hypothalamus.

Your answer: ☐

11. Neurons perform which of the following functions?

A. Transmitting and processing information.

B. Absorption and expunction.

C. Evolution and survival of the fittest.

D. None of the above.

Your answer:

12. The term converging operations is consistent with which of the following definitions?

A. A series of experiments conducted by the same discipline.

B. An assessment of test–retest reliability and external validity.

C. The lateralisation of the brain compensates for brain damage.

D. Numerous approaches working together to study phenomena at multiple levels.

Your answer:

Advanced level questions

13. The ability of the body to regulate its own natural state to restore balance is consistent with which of the following terms?

A. Goal-directed behaviour.

B. Homeostasis.

C. Transmission.

D. Psychopharmacology.

Your answer:

14. The tendency for living creatures to produce more than one offspring can be explained using which evolutionary principle?

A. Selective advantage.

B. Gene mutation.

C. Physiological evolution.

D. Sociocultural expansion.

Your answer:

15. Which of the following species do not feature in the evolution of humans?

    A. Homo erectus.

    B. Homo sapiens.

    C. Multituberculates.

    D. Neanderthals.

Your answer: ☐

16. Damage to which of the following regions frequently results in unilateral neglect?

    A. Frontal lobe.

    B. Left temporal lobe.

    C. Hypothalamus.

    D. Right parietal lobe.

Your answer: ☐

17. Neoteny facilitates the growth of larger brains but how does this occur?

    A. The maturation process is slowed.

    B. Genetic mutation occurs in the embryo.

    C. Selective variation between the mothers and fathers of the offspring.

    D. Mass extinction of species competing for resources.

Your answer: ☐

18. What is the name given to the pulse transmitted along neurons?

    A. Axon.

    B. Action potential.

    C. Dendrites.

    D. Agonist.

Your answer: ☐

19. Sensory homunculus is consistent with which of the following definitions?

A. Mapping of the body across the surface of the somatosensory cortex.

B. Re-uptake of neurotransmitters permitting conscious awareness.

C. Functionally restricted activity in the right hemisphere.

D. Deficits caused by frontal lobotomy.

Your answer: ☐

20. The degree to which certain characteristics shared by two people are due to genetics is consistent with which principle?

A. Mutation.

B. Reproductive success.

C. Natural selection.

D. Heritability.

Your answer: ☐

21. Which of the following is demonstrated in the physiology and anatomy of children?

A. Neural fixedness.

B. Neurotransmitter suppression.

C. Neuron plasticity.

D. All of the above.

Your answer: ☐

22. Which of the following would not be included in Melzack and Casey's (1968) dimensions of pain?

A. Universality of pain perception.

B. Perception of pain quality and intensity.

C. Cognitive appraisal of pain signals and source.

D. Motivation to withdraw from source.

Your answer: ☐

23. The ability of a cue which has been paired with a drug to mimic the drug's natural effects has been assigned which technical term?

A. Placebo.

B. Conditioned immune suppression effect.

C. Conditioned dualism.

D. Emergent properties.

Your answer:

24. Positron emission tomography exposes individuals to which substance?

A. Radioactively labelled glucose.

B. Magnetic fields.

C. X-ray.

D. None of the above.

Your answer:

25. Melzack and Wall (1965) proposed which of the following theories?

A. Placebo effects in depression.

B. Hedonic regulation of cravings.

C. Gate control theory of pain.

D. Garcia effects and aversion therapy.

Your answer:

26. Moniz won the Nobel Prize in Physiology or Medicine after developing which technique?

A. Magnetic resonance imaging.

B. Prefrontal leucotomy.

C. Functional magnetic resonance imaging.

D. Positron emission tomography.

Your answer:

Extended multiple-choice question

Match the following definitions with the disciplines listed below. Not all of the items will be consistent with the definitions and not all items can be used. Items can only be used once.

1. An approach which studies the neurological basis of behaviour and experience.

2. An approach which attempts to identify the cerebral structures associated with normal functioning by studying individuals with impaired functioning.

3. An approach which attempts to investigate and manipulate neural activity using various medications.

4. An approach which attempts to identify the correlates between physiology and psychological processes.

5. An approach which employs techniques such as fMRI to study the neural basis of cognition.

Optional items

A. Cognitive neuroscience

B. Comparative psychology

C. Evolutionary psychology

D. Parasympathetic psychology

E. Physiological psychology

F. Psychopharmacology

G. Psychophysiology

H. Neurophysiological psychology

I. Neuropsychology

J. Sympathetic psychology

Essay questions for Chapter 1

Once you have completed the MCQs you are ready to tackle the example essay questions below. You might like to select three or four topics and make notes on them. One way of doing this is to create a concept map. The first question has been done for you and you can see how the knowledge required links to some of the MCQs in this chapter.

1. Critically evaluate the methodologies and interdisciplinary links of biological psychology with reference to a minimum of two areas of study (e.g. memory and language).

2. To what extent have psychosurgery and neuroimaging contributed towards our understanding of mental health?

3. To what extent can reductionism contribute towards establishing a full and comprehensive account of human psychology?

4. Critically discuss the origins and contemporary practices of biological psychology with reference to philosophy, technology and experimentation.

5. Evaluate the insights into human cognition and behaviour which have been gained through psychopharmacology and neuropsychology.

6. Compare and contrast structuralist and functionalist contributions to contemporary biological psychology.

Chapter 1 essay question 1: concept map

Critically evaluate the methodologies and interdisciplinary links of biological psychology with reference to a minimum of two areas of study (e.g. memory and language).

The following concept map presents an example of how your responses to this question could be structured in a meaningful and comprehensive way. There are also links to specific questions in this chapter to guide your revision process. The applications of case studies, experiments, quasi-experiments, comparative studies, neuroimaging and neuropsychology are compared with reference to how these techniques can be used in several areas.

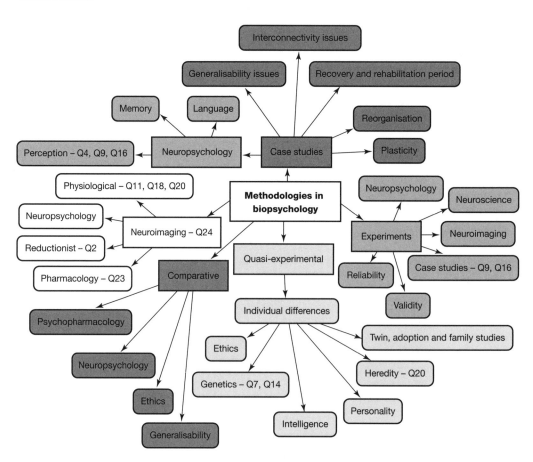

Chapter 2
The nervous system

This chapter provides questions relating to the nervous system. It includes topics such as the subdivisions of the nervous system in addition to the structures, functions, chemicals and measurement of the nervous system. It will test both your foundation and advanced knowledge of these topics. At the end of the chapter are several example essay questions and a sample concept map which may enable you to organise your thoughts during essay planning.

Select one answer for each question.

Foundation level questions

1. Which of the following fields of psychology employ biologically based methods during their investigations?

    A. Neuropsychology.

    B. Neuroscience.

    C. Health psychology.

    D. All of the above.

    Your answer: ☐

2. Which of these structures are parts of the central nervous system (CNS)?

    A. Brain and spinal cord.

    B. Muscles and tissue.

    C. Bones and ligaments.

    D. Stomach and adrenal gland.

    Your answer: ☐

3. What is the full name given to the PNS?

    A. Periphery nervous system.

    B. Peripheral nervous system.

    C. Parallel nervous system.

    D. Pedagogical neuron system.

Your answer: ☐

4. What is the function of nociceptive neurons?

    A. Detecting and absorbing vitamin D.

    B. Transmitting signals from the central nervous system.

    C. Detecting tissue damage at their tips.

    D. Conveying visual information along the cranial nerves.

Your answer: ☐

5. Cranial nerves are found in which of the following areas?

    A. Above the neck, including from the eyes, ears and nose.

    B. Only leading from the optic nerves.

    C. Only leading from the ears.

    D. Only leading from the mouth.

Your answer: ☐

6. Transmission of which of the following would result in the release of a neurotransmitter?

    A. Motor cells.

    B. Sensory cells.

    C. Receptors.

    D. Action potentials.

Your answer: ☐

7. What is the function of an artificial chemical within the antagonist category?

   A. Blocking the effects of a neurotransmitter by occupying the receptors.

   B. Mimicking a neurotransmitter.

   C. Repairing faults in the synaptic gaps.

   D. Facilitating neural plasticity and regrowth.

Your answer: ☐

8. What response is produced by the neurotransmitter dopamine?

   A. Pain.

   B. Sadness.

   C. Pleasure.

   D. Fear.

Your answer: ☐

9. Adrenalin and noradrenalin function as which of the following?

   A. Hormone.

   B. Neurotransmitter and hormone.

   C. Neurotransmitter.

   D. Sensory homunculus.

Your answer: ☐

10. Luria (1973) identified that which cerebral region is associated with planning?

   A. Frontal lobes.

   B. Temporal lobes.

   C. Amygdala.

   D. Hippocampus.

Your answer: ☐

11. Which of the following is a primary difference between the parasympathetic and sympathetic nervous systems?

A. Parasympathetic is inhibitory, sympathetic is excitatory.

B. Parasympathetic is excitatory, sympathetic is inhibitory.

C. Parasympathetic is in the CNS, sympathetic is in the autonomic nervous system (ANS).

D. Parasympathetic is in the ANS, sympathetic is in the CNS.

Your answer: ☐

12. Which of the following are associated with the stress response?

A. Central nervous system.

B. Sympathetic nervous system.

C. Immune system and adrenal gland.

D. All of the above.

Your answer: ☐

Advanced level questions

13. Which of the following are produced by Schwann cells?

A. Myelin in the CNS.

B. Myelin in the PNS.

C. Noradrenalin in the PNS.

D. Serotonin in the PNS.

Your answer: ☐

14. Acetylcholine terminates postsynaptic potentials by which function?

A. Blocking receptor cells.

B. Blocking terminal buttons.

C. Destroying molecules of a neurotransmitter.

D. Promoting re-uptake.

Your answer: ☐

15. Which of the following form the meninges?

  A. Dura mater.

  B. Arachnoid membrane.

  C. Pia mater.

  D. All of the above.

Your answer: ☐

16. Apoptosis refers to which phenomenon?

  A. Death of a cell due to genetic mechanisms triggered by chemical signals.

  B. Cells rapidly grow outwards in the ventricular zone.

  C. Cells divide and multiply in the central nervous system.

  D. Migration of twin cells from the ventricular zone to the brain.

Your answer: ☐

17. Which of the following structures receive information concerning taste?

  A. Lateral fissure.

  B. Insular cortex.

  C. Central sulcus.

  D. Calcarine fissure.

Your answer: ☐

18. Which structures are located within the temporal lobe?

  A. Visual and somatosensory association cortex.

  B. Motor and visual association cortex.

  C. Auditory and visual association cortex.

  D. Somatosensory and motor association cortex.

Your answer: ☐

19. The limbic system has been associated with which of the following?

   A. Emotion and motivation.

   B. Learning.

   C. Memory.

   D. All of the above.

Your answer: ☐

20. What is the alternative name given to the midbrain?

   A. Mesencephalon.

   B. Telencephalon.

   C. Metencephalon.

   D. Diencephalon.

Your answer: ☐

21. Which of the following can be used to study a membrane's potential?

   A. Oscilloscope.

   B. Magnetic resonance imaging.

   C. Lesions.

   D. Case studies in neuropsychology.

Your answer: ☐

22. Movement is contolled by which two groups of descending tracts in the brain?

   A. Dorsal and lateral.

   B. Medial and ventral.

   C. Lateral and ventromedial.

   D. Caudal and dorsal.

Your answer: ☐

23. What is the term given to a long-term increase in the excitability of a neuron caused by repeated exposure?

   A. Population EPSP.

   B. Fight or flight.

   C. Conduction aphasia.

   D. Long-term potentiation.

Your answer: ☐

Extended multiple-choice question

Complete the following paragraph using the items listed overleaf. Not all of the items will be consistent with the paragraph and not all items can be used.

The human nervous system is a complex organisation consisting of several branches and complex neural pathways. For example, the _____ incorporates the brain and spinal cord and is responsible for several regulatory processes and cognition. In contrast, the _____ consists of all of the nerves and ganglia located beyond the central nervous system. This system functions primarily as a connection to the central nervous system although some of the pathways, such as the _____, can function independently. The PNS can also be differentiated by two prominent overarching systems. The _____ consists of efferent nerves and is responsible for controlling voluntary movement. In contrast the _____ consists of both afferent and efferent neurons and primarily operates beyond consciousness.

(For optional items see overleaf)

Optional items

A. autonomic nervous system

B. associative nervous system

C. dorsal nervous system

D. enteric nervous system

E. central nervous system (CNS)

F. centralised peripheral nervous system (CPNS)

G. peripheral nervous system (PNS)

H. respiratory nervous system

I. somatic nervous system

J. ventral nervous system (VNS)

Essay questions for Chapter 2

Once you have completed the MCQs you are ready to tackle the example essay questions below. You might like to select three or four topics and make notes on them. One way of doing this is to create a concept map. The first question has been done for you and you can see how the knowledge required links to some of the MCQs in this chapter.

1. Compare and contrast the structure and functions of the central and peripheral nervous systems.

2. To what extent has biopsychology contributed towards understanding the nature of the human nervous system?

3. Critically evaluate the benefits and limitations of methodologies used in biopsychology with reference to studying the central and peripheral nervous systems.

4. Critically discuss and evaluate the modular view of the central nervous system with reference to a minimum of two areas of research (e.g. memory and learning).

5. To what extent has biopsychology successfully united science, physiology, neuroscience, neuropsychology and traditional psychological experimentation?

6. Critically evaluate the role of the limbic system in human experience and behaviour.

7. Compare and contrast the insights drawn from research investigating the nervous system in its intact and damaged states.

Chapter 2 essay question 1: concept map

Compare and contrast the structure and functions of the central and peripheral nervous systems.

The following concept map presents an example of how responses to this question could be structured in a meaningful and comprehensive way. The structures and functions of the central and peripheral nervous system are compared and contrasted with specific links to relevant questions in this chapter to guide your revision process.

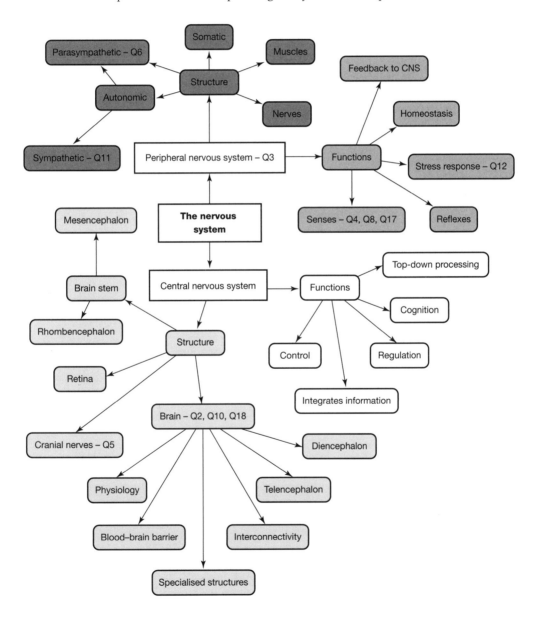

Chapter 3:
Sensory systems I – touch, temperature and pain

This chapter provides questions relating to the sensory systems which facilitate the perception of touch, temperature and pain. It includes topics such as schools of thought, the scope of the subject, key terms and concepts, methodological considerations and prominent milestones in research. It will test both your foundation and advanced knowledge of these topics. At the end of the chapter are several example essay questions and a sample concept map which may enable you to organise your thoughts during essay planning.

Select one answer for each question.

Foundation level questions

1. Sensory transduction is the term assigned to which of the following processes?

    A. Translation of physical event into an electrical signal by sensory receptors.

    B. Translation of action potentials into chemicals in synapses.

    C. Translation of electrical signals into cortical activity by the central nervous system.

    D. Translation of physical events into chemical reactions in neurons.

    Your answer: ☐

2. The tendency for a neuron to be unresponsive to a steady stream of information is known by which term?

    A. Desensitisation.

    B. Adaptation.

    C. Tolerance.

    D. Resting potential.

    Your answer: ☐

3. Which of the following are located near the surface of the skin and facilitate the sense of touch?

   A. Interneurons.

   B. Inter cranial neurons.

   C. Capillaries.

   D. Somatosensory neurons.

   Your answer: ☐

4. Kinesthesia is the term assigned to which of the following somatosenses?

   A. Perception of the body's movement.

   B. Perception of pain.

   C. Perception of temperature.

   D. Perception of touch.

   Your answer: ☐

5. Which of the following contributes towards the greater sensitivity observed at the centre of the sensory receptive field?

   A. Neurotransmitters.

   B. Blood flow.

   C. Density of receptor branches.

   D. Glucose metabolism.

   Your answer: ☐

6. What is the primary function of nociceptive neurons?

   A. Detecting changes in temperature.

   B. Detecting real or threatened tissue damage.

   C. Detecting changes in pressure.

   D. Detecting changes in general sensory pathways.

   Your answer: ☐

7. In which cerebral structure is information from the somatosensory neurons processed?

A. Thalamus.

B. Amygdala.

C. Occipital cortex.

D. Hippocampus.

Your answer: ☐

8. Which of the following describes a commonality between pain and temperature sensitive neurons?

A. Both transmit information from the PNS to muscle via the spinal cord.

B. Both transmit information from the PNS to CNS without the spinal cord.

C. Both transmit information from the CNS via cranial nerves.

D. Both transmit information from the PNS to CNS via the spinal cord.

Your answer: ☐

9. Which of the following structures are found in glabrous skin?

A. Ruffini corpuscles.

B. Pacinian corpuscles.

C. Meissner's corpuscles.

D. All of the above.

Your answer: ☐

10. Which type of cell is receptive to nociceptive neurons according to the gate theory of pain?

A. R-cells.

B. P-cells.

C. T-cells.

D. D-cells.

Your answer: ☐

11. Enkephalin is a naturally produced chemical in which of the following categories?

   A. Opioid.

   B. Stimulant.

   C. Depressant.

   D. Hallucinogen.

Your answer:

12. Phantom limb pain is an example of which of the following?

   A. Bottom-up processing and primacy of PNS.

   B. Top-down processing and active role of the brain.

   C. The brain cannot generate pain sensations.

   D. Pain can be generated by the PNS without corresponding activity in the brain.

Your answer:

Advanced level questions

13. Which of the following is true in regard to temperature?

   A. Perceptions of temperature are relative except at the extremes.

   B. Perceptions of temperature are universal at all levels.

   C. Perceptions of temperature are relative at extremes.

   D. Perceptions of temperature are produced solely by the CNS.

Your answer:

14. Damage to the insular cortex can cause which of the following?

   A. No perception of pain but automatic withdrawal from the cause.

   B. No perception of pain and failure to withdraw from the cause.

   C. Perception of pain after automatic withdrawal.

   D. Perception of pain but no recognition that it is harmful or withdrawal from the cause.

Your answer:

15. Spray (1986) proposed that which mechanism is responsible for transmitting signals relating to coolness?

   A. Sodium chloride pump.

   B. Sodium potassium pump.

   C. Sodium amytal pump.

   D. None of the above.

Your answer: ☐

16. Dykes (1983) identified that the primary and secondary somatosensory cortical areas can be divided into how many maps of the body?

   A. 5–10.

   B. 10–15.

   C. 0–5.

   D. 15–20.

Your answer: ☐

17. Patients MT and EC demonstrated which pattern of impairment associated with tactile agnosia?

   A. Objects and drawings seen but not felt.

   B. Objects recognised but not felt.

   C. Objects and drawings felt but not seen.

   D. Drawings recognised but not felt.

Your answer: ☐

18. Which cerebral regions are associated with the pathway responsible for the immediate emotional component of pain?

   A. Anterior cingulate cortex and insular cortex.

   B. Prefrontal cortex and thalamus.

   C. Thalamus and insular cortex.

   D. Anterior cingulate cortex and prefrontal cortex.

Your answer: ☐

19. Ostrowsky et al. (2002) observed that stimulation of the insular cortex caused which of the following?

   A. Feelings of pain and burning.

   B. Activation in the prefrontal cortex.

   C. Feelings of cold but no pain.

   D. No effect.

Your answer: ☐

20. Melzack and Wall (1965) proposed that nerve fibres transmit signals to which of the following?

   A. ON and OFF receptors in the retina.

   B. Inhibitory and transmission cells in the dorsal horn.

   C. Hidden and output units in connectionist representations.

   D. Cranial nerves and synapses located near the cerebellum.

Your answer: ☐

21. What term is assigned to the inhibition of motor neurons?

   A. Re-synthesis inhibition.

   B. Interneuron inhibition.

   C. Recurrent collateral inhibition.

   D. Isomorphic inhibition.

Your answer: ☐

22. Which difficulty do people with apraxia experience?

   A. Completing voluntary movements when requested out of context.

   B. Perceiving pain at extreme temperatures.

   C. Perceiving touch on their left side.

   D. Demonstrating the startle response and automatic reflexes.

Your answer: ☐

23. Which of the following areas are associated with the secondary motor cortex?

   A. Premotor cortex.

   B. Primary motor cortex.

   C. Cingulate motor cortex.

   D. All of the above.

Your answer: ☐

24. Astereognosia refers to deficits in which of the following?

   A. Identifying sources of pain.

   B. Identifying objects by touch.

   C. Identifying bodily positions.

   D. Identifying sharpness.

Your answer: ☐

Extended multiple-choice question

Complete the following paragraph using the items listed opposite. Not all of the items will be consistent with the paragraph and not all items can be used. Items can only be used once.

The somatosensory system is a complex and diverse aspect of the human organism which monitors and responds to information obtained from _____. Indeed, Pinel's (2003) model of the system incorporates hierarchical, cascading and parallel processing between the central nervous system and _____. For example, the _____ transmits information to the secondary motor cortex, primary motor cortex, brain stem motor nuclei and spinal motor circuits. However, transmission of information also occurs within and between these other structures via _____. Furthermore, information is transmitted from muscles and the peripheral nervous system to each level of the central nervous system via _____. This demonstrates the complex and vital nature of this system.

Optional items

A. association cortex

B. bodily senses

C. chemical senses

D. cerebellum

E. descending motor circuits

F. electrolytes

G. feedback circuits

H. mitosis

I. parasympathetic

J. peripheral nervous system

Essay questions for Chapter 3

Once you have completed the MCQs you are ready to tackle the example essay questions below. You might like to select three or four topics and make notes on them. One way of doing this is to create a concept map. The first question has been done for you and you can see how the knowledge required links to some of the MCQs in this chapter.

1. To what extent is knowledge of the somatosensory systems based on biological rather than psychological factors? Evaluate the evidence and identify the strengths and limitations of each approach.

2. Critically evaluate the gate theory of pain with reference to both theory and research.

3. Compare and contrast the sensory systems responsible for detecting touch, temperature and pain.

4. To what extent has the study of intact and impaired sensory systems contributed towards the understanding of touch and pain pathways?

5. Evaluate the benefits and limitations of research investigating the nature, scope and functioning of the somatosensory systems.

6. To what extent can the somatosensory systems be considered to be independent of other sensory systems?

7. Evaluate the top-down and bottom-up accounts of the somatosensory system.

8. Critically discuss the claim that perceptions of temperature are relative rather than absolute.

Chapter 3 essay question 1: concept map

To what extent is knowledge of the somatosensory systems based on biological rather than psychological factors? Evaluate the evidence and identify the strengths and limitations of each approach.

The following concept map presents an example of how your responses to this question could be structured in a meaningful and comprehensive way. There are also links to specific questions in this chapter to guide your revision process. The main influences of biological and psychological factors in somatosensory systems are compared and contrasted with specific examples from the chapter. The techniques, strengths and limitations of these approaches are also incorporated into the concept map.

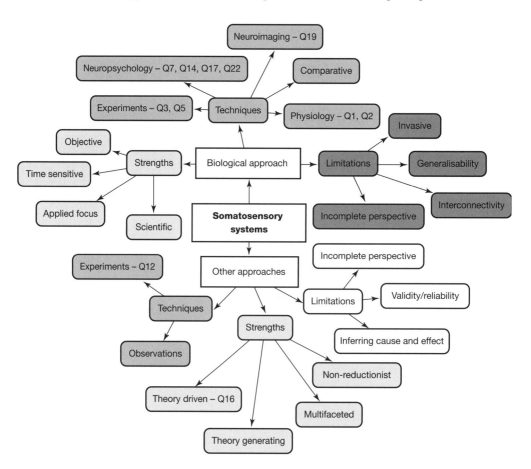

Chapter 4
Sensory systems II – sight, sound, taste and smell

This chapter provides questions relating to the sensory systems which facilitate the perception of sight, sound, taste and smell. It includes topics such as schools of thought, the scope of the subject, key terms and concepts, methodological considerations and prominent milestones in research. It will test both your foundation and advanced knowledge of these topics. At the end of the chapter are several example essay questions and a sample concept map which may enable you to organise your thoughts during essay planning.

Select one answer for each question.

Foundation level questions

1. What are the alternative names for the external ear and eardrum respectively?

    A. Pinna and tympanic membrane.

    B. Malleus and pinna.

    C. Ossicles and tympanic membrane.

    D. Incus and oval window.

    Your answer:

2. The organ of Corti transmits auditory information to the brain through which of the following?

    A. Cilium.

    B. Nociceptive neuron.

    C. Cochlear nerve.

    D. Tectorial.

    Your answer:

3. Which neurotransmitter is present at the afferent synapses in the olivocochlear bundle?

A. Acetylcholine.

B. Glutamate.

C. Serotonin.

D. Dopamine.

Your answer: ☐

4. Which substance is secreted at the efferent terminal buttons in the olivocochlear bundle?

A. Glutamate.

B. Serotonin.

C. Dopamine.

D. Acetylcholine.

Your answer: ☐

5. The cochlear nucleus is located in which of the following structures?

A. Medulla.

B. Thalamus.

C. Pituitary.

D. Temporal lobe.

Your answer: ☐

6. The primary auditory cortex consists of how many regions?

A. Six.

B. Three.

C. Two.

D. Five.

Your answer: ☐

7. The dorsal stream of the auditory cortex terminates in which structure?

    A. Posterior parietal cortex.

    B. Anterior parietal cortex.

    C. Parabelt region.

    D. Inferior colliculus.

Your answer: ☐

8. Which of the terms below reflects the relationship between the cortex and basilar membrane?

    A. Lateral lemniscus.

    B. Fundamental frequency.

    C. Phase difference.

    D. Tonotopic representation.

Your answer: ☐

9. The olfactory epithelium is tissue covering which of the following?

    A. Olfactory bulb.

    B. Cribriform plate.

    C. Olfactory glomerulus.

    D. Nucleus raphe magnus.

Your answer: ☐

10. What is the functional role of vergence movement?

    A. To ensure all information from the visual scene reaches the optical nerve.

    B. To maintain the image of a moving object.

    C. To ensure an image falls in an identical area on each retina.

    D. To facilitate the process of accommodation.

Your answer: ☐

11. The rods and cones in the retina are collectively known as which of the following?

A. Photoreceptors.

B. Ganglion.

C. Bipolar cells.

D. Fovea.

Your answer:

Advanced level questions

12. Which of the following items are layers in the dorsal lateral geniculate nucleus?

A. Magnocellular.

B. Parvocellular.

C. Koniocellular.

D. All of the above.

Your answer:

13. Schiller, Sandell and Maunsell (1986) injected monkeys with amino phosphonobutyrate to achieve which of the following?

A. Deactivation of taste sensations.

B. Hypersensitivity to unpleasant odours.

C. Impairment of contrast sensitivity.

D. Reversal of congenital blindness.

Your answer:

14. To what does the trichromatic theory refer?

A. Colour vision.

B. Depth perception.

C. Pitch perception.

D. Components of gustation.

Your answer:

15. Individuals with the condition tritanopia demonstrate which pattern of impairment?

   A. Impaired vision for hues with long wavelengths but see in shades of blue.

   B. Impaired vision for hues with short wavelengths but see in green and red.

   C. Impaired colour vision and see in black and white.

   D. Impaired vision for hues with short wavelengths but see in yellow and blue.

Your answer: ☐

16. Additional processing of the wavelength of light is performed by which structure before being transmitted to the visual association cortex?

   A. Striate cortex.

   B. Hippocampus.

   C. Fusiform.

   D. Frontal lobe.

Your answer: ☐

17. Stereopsis is a product of which of the following?

   A. Sine-wave grating.

   B. Retinal disparity.

   C. Protanopia.

   D. Deuteranopia.

Your answer: ☐

18. Individuals with blindsight demonstrate which pattern of impairment?

   A. Inability to reach for objects which are not consciously seen in the unimpaired visual field.

   B. Inability to see objects in the left visual field.

   C. Inability to see objects in the right visual field.

   D. Ability to reach for objects which are not consciously seen in the impaired visual field.

Your answer: ☐

19. In which cerebral structure does recognition of patterns and the identification of objects typically occur?

    A. Inferior temporal cortex.

    B. Frontal lobe.

    C. Medulla.

    D. Amygdala.

Your answer: ☐

20. Prosopagnosia is a form of which condition?

    A. Apraxia.

    B. Dyslexia.

    C. Visual agnosia.

    D. Anomia.

Your answer: ☐

21. The chorda tympani transmit information for which sensory system?

    A. Olfactory.

    B. Gustatory.

    C. Tactile.

    D. Visual.

Your answer: ☐

22. What are the five qualities detected by the taste receptors?

    A. Bitterness, heat, sweetness, sourness and umami.

    B. Cold, saltiness, sweetness, sourness and bitterness.

    C. Sweetness, heat, cold, bitterness and saltiness.

    D. Umami, saltiness, sweetness, sourness and bitterness.

Your answer: ☐

Extended multiple-choice question

Match the following definitions with the appropriate term listed below. Not all of the items will be consistent with the definitions and not all items can be used. Items can only be used once.

1. This term is assigned to the system consisting of semicircular canals and receptor organs in the inner ear.

2. This term is assigned to the sensory system which is responsible for taste.

3. This term is assigned to the sensory system which is responsible for smell.

4. This term is assigned to the dendrites of mitral cells and the terminal buttons of axons in the sensory system responsible for smell.

5. This term is applied to the taste sensation produced by glutamate.

Optional items

A. Audition

B. Gustation

C. Insertional plate

D. Malleus

E. Olfaction

F. Olfactory glomerulus

G. Parabelt

H. Tectorial membrane

I. Umami

J. Vestibular

Essay questions for Chapter 4

Once you have completed the MCQs you are ready to tackle the example essay questions below. You might like to select three or four topics and make notes on them. One way of doing this is to create a concept map. The first question has been done for you and you can see how the knowledge required links to some of the MCQs in this chapter.

1. Evaluate the insights provided by studies investigating impaired bodily senses and normal functioning.

2. Compare and contrast a minimum of two sensory systems from the options of taste, smell, sight and sound with reference to both anatomical pathways and experimental research.

3. To what extent are the gustatory and olfactory sensory systems co-dependent on each other?

4. Critically discuss the roles of the peripheral and central nervous systems in determining vision and audition.

5. To what extent can vision be considered to be a product of top-down and bottom-up processing?

6. Evaluate the role of neurotransmitters in regard to the bodily and chemical senses with reference to a minimum of two senses.

7. Critically discuss and evaluate research investigating face perception with reference to both normal and damaged visual pathways.

8. To what extent has biopsychology contributed towards the understanding of audition and olfaction?

Chapter 4 essay question 1: concept map

Evaluate the insights provided by studies investigating impaired bodily senses and normal functioning.

The following concept map presents an example of how your responses to this question could be structured in a meaningful and comprehensive way. There are also links to specific questions in this chapter to guide your revision process. The methodologies, strengths and limitations for studying bodily senses are critically reviewed with specific examples from the chapter.

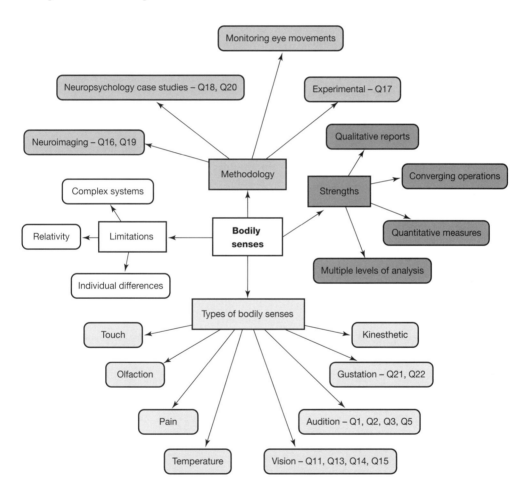

Chapter 5
Motivation

This chapter provides questions relating to the biological and psychological factors associated with motivation. It includes topics such as schools of thought, the scope of the subject (for example, hunger, health, sleep and reproduction), key terms and concepts, methodological considerations and prominent milestones in research. It will test both your foundation and advanced knowledge of these topics. At the end of the chapter are several example essay questions and a sample concept map which may enable you to organise your thoughts during essay planning.

Select one answer for each question.

Foundation level questions

1. Which of the following do not have a biological motivation?

    A. Sleep and hunger.

    B. Reproduction and appraisal of stimuli.

    C. Fight or flight and drug addiction.

    D. None of the above.

    Your answer: ☐

2. Which of the following hormones is not influential in male reproductive behaviour?

    A. Prolactin.

    B. Oxytocin.

    C. Estrogen.

    D. Testosterone.

    Your answer: ☐

3. Which of the following is the term assigned to the chemical which, when secreted from one animal, can influence the behaviour or physiology of another animal?

   A. Hormone.

   B. Pheromone.

   C. Neurotransmitter.

   D. Action potentials.

   Your answer: ☐

4. Which of the following can be used to record activity during sleep?

   A. Electroencephalography (EEG).

   B. Electromyography (EMG).

   C. Electrooculography (EOG).

   D. All of the above.

   Your answer: ☐

5. In which state are alpha waves typically recorded?

   A. Relaxation.

   B. Arousal.

   C. Anger.

   D. Fear.

   Your answer: ☐

6. Which of the following occurs during early slow wave sleep and rapid eye movement (REM) sleep?

   A. Delta activity.

   B. Theta activity.

   C. Alpha activity.

   D. Beta activity.

   Your answer: ☐

7. The 90-minute basic rest–activity cycle is controlled by which structure?

   A. Hippocampus.

   B. Thalamus.

   C. Caudal brain stem.

   D. Medulla.

   Your answer: ☐

8. Sleep apnoea is characterised by which of the following behaviours?

   A. Cessation of breathing while sleeping.

   B. Inability to sleep.

   C. Sleepwalking.

   D. Sleep talking.

   Your answer: ☐

9. Lisk, Pretlow and Friedman (1969) identified that which chemical facilitates nest building?

   A. Testosterone.

   B. Progesterone.

   C. Serotonin.

   D. Acetylcholine.

   Your answer: ☐

10. The destruction of hypocretin causes which of the following conditions?

   A. Insomnia.

   B. Sleep apnoea.

   C. Impulsivity.

   D. Narcolepsy.

   Your answer: ☐

11. Peptide YY is produced after a meal in proportion to which of the following?

   A. Calories.

   B. Sugars.

   C. Salts.

   D. Weights.

Your answer: ☐

Advanced level questions

12. Horne (1978) observed that sleep may serve which function?

   A. Permitting the body to rest and maintaining healthy physical functions.

   B. Permitting the body and brain to rest but only maintaining healthy physical functions.

   C. Permitting the brain to rest and maintaining healthy cognitive functions.

   D. Permitting the body and brain to rest but only maintaining healthy cognitive functions.

Your answer: ☐

13. Insulin is produced by which organ?

   A. Pancreas.

   B. Liver.

   C. Kidney.

   D. Stomach.

Your answer: ☐

14. Which of the following contain a neurotransmitter which is not associated with sleep?

   A. Acetylcholine and hypocretin.

   B. Serotonin and histamine.

   C. Histamine and dopamine.

   D. Norepinephrine and serotonin.

Your answer: ☐

15. What term is applied to a dramatic fall in the levels of fatty acids available to cells which may cause feelings of hunger?

A. Lipoprivation.

B. Glucoprivation.

C. Isomorphism.

D. Metabolism.

Your answer: ☐

16. McClintock (1971) observed synchronisation of which of the following?

A. Homeostasis patterns in human family groups.

B. Lifecycles of rats housed in the same laboratory.

C. Circadian rhythms among all male ape populations.

D. Menstrual cycles among women at an all-female college.

Your answer: ☐

17. Cutting the connections between the brain stem and which area abolishes maternal behaviour?

A. Sexual dimorphic nucleus.

B. Medial preoptic area.

C. Periaqueductal grey matter.

D. Vomeronasal organ.

Your answer: ☐

18. What term is applied to the type of thirst caused by increased pressure of the interstitial fluid compared to the intracellular fluid?

A. Osmometric.

B. Volumetric.

C. Angiotensin.

D. Glucoprivation.

Your answer: ☐

19. Fava et al. (1989) argued that anorexia and bulimia are characterised by changes in which substances respectively?

   A. 5-HT in anorexia and NE in bulimia.

   B. Dopamine in anorexia and serotonin in bulimia.

   C. Adrenaline in bulimia and dopamine in anorexia.

   D. NE in anorexia and 5-HT in bulimia.

Your answer: ☐

20. Cholecystokinin appears to send which form of signal to the brain through the vagus nerve?

   A. Satiety.

   B. Thirst.

   C. Arousal.

   D. Tiredness.

Your answer: ☐

21. Saxena et al. (1998) identified that reducing the activity in which cerebral structures reduced the symptoms of obsessive compulsive disorder?

   A. Amygdala and thalamus.

   B. Caudate nucleus and orbitofrontal cortex.

   C. Hippocampus and caudate nucleus.

   D. All of the above.

Your answer: ☐

22. What are the primary sites influenced by alcohol consumption and what function does it serve at these sites?

   A. GABA receptors as an indirect agonist and NMDA receptors as an indirect antagonist.

   B. GABA receptors as a direct agonist and NMDA receptors as an indirect antagonist.

   C. GABA receptors as a direct antagonist and NMDA receptors as a direct agonist.

   D. None of the above.

Your answer: ☐

23. Cloninger (1987) argued that steady and binge drinkers were influenced by which factors respectively?

    A. Steady drinkers and binge drinkers both influenced by environment.

    B. Steady drinkers and binge drinkers both influenced by physiology and genetics.

    C. Steady drinkers influenced by heredity, binge drinkers by heredity and environment.

    D. Steady drinkers influenced by environment, binge drinkers by heredity.

Your answer: ☐

Extended multiple-choice question

Match the following definitions with the terms below. Not all of the items will be consistent with the definitions and not all items can be used. Items can only be used once.

1. A condition characterised by excessive body mass index which places the individual at risk of health problems, specifically heart disease and stroke. ☐

2. A condition characterised by sporadic binging and purging which can harm the digestive tract. ☐

3. A condition characterised by under-consumption, serious health complications and an emaciated appearance. ☐

4. A condition characterised by the uncontrollable, sporadic need to sleep. Also often categorised by cataplexy, sleep paralysis and hypnagogic hallucinations. ☐

5. A condition characterised by an inability to sleep despite an often strong motivation to do so. ☐

Optional items

    A. Addiction

    B. Anorexia nervosa

    C. Apraxia

    D. Bulimia

E. Hypothalamic impairment

F. Insomnia

G. Korsakoff's syndrome

H. Narcolepsy

I. Obesity

J. REM sleep deprivation

Essay questions for Chapter 5

Once you have completed the MCQs you are ready to tackle the example essay questions below. You might like to select three or four topics and make notes on them. One way of doing this is to create a concept map. The first question has been done for you and you can see how the knowledge required links to some of the MCQs in this chapter.

1. Critically discuss the biological influences exerted on at least two forms of motivation (for example, sleep and hunger).

2. Compare and contrast biological factors associated with substance abuse and eating disorders.

3. To what extent has physiology and neuroimaging contributed towards the understanding of the normal motivation for sleep and the factors associated with sleep disorders?

4. Compare and contrast the biological and cognitive approaches to studying motivation.

5. Evaluate the methodologies available to study human motivation from a biological perspective.

6. To what extent is the motivation for reproduction produced by solely biological factors?

7. Critically discuss the claim that research with non-human animals has contributed nothing towards understanding human motivation.

8. Critically discuss biological and environmental influences on human motivation with reference to both normal and maladaptive behaviours.

Chapter 5 essay question 1: concept map

Critically discuss the biological influences exerted on at least two forms of motivation (for example sleep and hunger).

The following concept map represents an example of how your responses to this question could be structured in a meaningful and comprehensive way. There are also links to specific questions in this chapter to guide your revision process. The biological influences on the motivations of hunger, sleep and addiction are compared and contrasted using examples from the chapter and alternative non-biological factors.

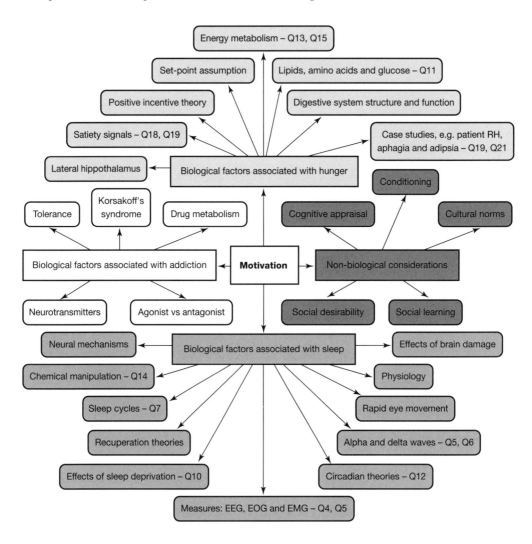

Chapter 6
Emotion

This chapter provides questions relating to the biological and psychological factors associated with emotion. It includes topics such as schools of thought, key terms and concepts, normal emotional responses, maladaptive emotional responses, methodological considerations and prominent milestones in research. It will test both your foundation and advanced knowledge of these topics. At the end of the chapter are several example essay questions and a sample concept map which may enable you to organise your thoughts during essay planning.

Select one answer for each question.

Foundation level questions

1. Which of the following is consistent with the James-Lange theory?

    A. Behaviour is a direct response elicited by stimuli.

    B. Physiology is a direct response elicited by stimuli.

    C. Emotional responses are produced by feedback from behaviour and physiology.

    D. All of the above.

    Your answer: ☐

2. Which of the following individuals argued that facial expressions were innate and evolved responses?

    A. Jones.

    B. Darwin.

    C. Vergness.

    D. Kaye.

    Your answer: ☐

3. Frijda et al. (1989) argued emotions serve which of the following functions?

    A. Guiding primary appraisal.

    B. Guiding secondary appraisal.

    C. Promoting action readiness.

    D. Determining valence of stimuli.

Your answer: ☐

4. Which of the following conditions demonstrates examples of when emotional processing and responses are impaired or maladaptive?

    A. Autism.

    B. Depression.

    C. Obsessive compulsive disorder.

    D. All of the above.

Your answer: ☐

5. Which of these cerebral structures relay emotional information according to LeDoux's (1992, 1996) fast circuit?

    A. Thalamus and amygdala.

    B. Hypothalamus and hippocampus.

    C. Left temporal lobe and orbitofrontal cortex.

    D. Thalamus and prefrontal cortex.

Your answer: ☐

6. Neuropsychology patient DR experienced difficulties processing emotion after damage to which cerebral structure?

    A. Primary motor cortex.

    B. Left and right amygdala.

    C. Left parietal lobe.

    D. Corpus callosum.

Your answer: ☐

7. How many regions in the amygdala have been associated with the fear response?

    A. Eight.

    B. None.

    C. Three.

    D. Five.

Your answer:

8. Rosenthal (1971) argued that major affective disorders were more prevalent in which of the following?

    A. Eastern cultures.

    B. Western cultures.

    C. Individuals with a family history of affective disorders.

    D. Women and young girls.

Your answer:

9. Hess (1950) identified that electrical stimulation of which cerebral structure produced irritability, alertness, arousal and aggression in cats?

    A. Hypothalamus.

    B. Hippocampus.

    C. Hindbrain.

    D. Cerebellum.

Your answer:

10. Prenatal androgenisation increases which of the following responses?

    A. Passivity.

    B. Aggression.

    C. Sexual arousal.

    D. Fear.

Your answer:

11. The treatment of bipolar depression using lithium has which of the following limitations?

   A. Low therapeutic index (the difference between effective dose and overdose).

   B. Side effects including hand tremors, nausea, poor motor coordination and confusion.

   C. Tendency for patients to terminate medication.

   D. All of the above.

   Your answer: ☐

12. Phineas Gage experienced damage to which cerebral structure associated with aggression?

   A. Orbitofrontal cortex.

   B. Cerebellum.

   C. Olfactory cortex.

   D. None of the above.

   Your answer: ☐

13. Which of the following can be used to stimulate the cortex or infuse chemicals in the brain?

   A. Positron emission tomography.

   B. Magnetic resonance imaging.

   C. Cannula electrodes.

   D. Lesions.

   Your answer: ☐

Advanced level questions

14. How many cerebral routes to anxiety did Gray (1982) initially identify?

    A. Two.

    B. Four.

    C. One.

    D. Six.

Your answer: ☐

15. Low levels of the serotonin metabolite 5-HIAA is associated with which of the following states in rhesus monkeys and humans?

    A. Passivity and dismissive gestures.

    B. Anger and aggression.

    C. Sadness and depression.

    D. Fear and depression.

Your answer: ☐

16. LeDoux (1988, 1995) identified that removal of which structure impaired conditioned responses, changes in blood pressure and the freezing response respectively?

    A. Central nucleus, caudal periaqueductal grey matter and lateral hypothalamus.

    B. Lateral hypothalamus, central nucleus and caudal periaqueductal grey matter.

    C. Central nucleus, lateral hypothalamus and caudal periaqueductal grey matter.

    D. Caudal periaqueductal grey matter, central nucleus and lateral hypothalamus.

Your answer: ☐

17. Vogel et al. (1990) observed that all medications which suppress REM sleep have which other function?

    A. Antipsychotic.

    B. Antidepressant.

    C. Anxiolytic.

    D. None of the above.

Your answer: ☐

18. Beauregard, Lévesque and Bourgouin (2001) observed which pattern of activation when instructing male participants to inhibit their emotional responses to erotic films?

A. Parts of the limbic system and prefrontal cortex were activated.

B. Parts of the limbic system were activated but the prefrontal cortex was not.

C. There was no change in activation to that observed when participants reacted normally.

D. The limbic system was not activated but the prefrontal cortex was activated.

Your answer: ☐

19. Bean (1982) identified that lesioning which of the following regions eradicated inter-male aggression among mice?

A. Vomeronasal nerve.

B. Amygdala.

C. Hypothalamus.

D. Limbic system.

Your answer: ☐

20. Ekman and Friesen (1971) conducted which type of study to investigate the evolutionary theory of facial expressions?

A. Cross-cultural.

B. Neuroimaging.

C. Prevalence study.

D. Twin study.

Your answer: ☐

21. The MAO inhibitor iproniazid increases the release of which of the following?

A. Noradrenalin, serotonin and androgen.

B. Lipids, dopamine and serotonin.

C. Serotonin, dopamine and norepinephrine.

D. Beta waves, alpha waves and norepinephrine.

Your answer: ☐

22. Tricyclic antidepressants alleviate symptoms of depression by which function?

    A. Antagonist of serotonin.

    B. Antagonist of dopamine.

    C. Facilitating the re-uptake of 5-HT.

    D. Inhibiting the re-uptake of 5-HT and norepinephrine.

Your answer: ☐

23. Fischer et al. (1998) observed which pattern of cerebral activation during the unexpected panic attack of a participant?

    A. Decreased activity in the right orbitofrontal cortex.

    B. Decreased activity in anterior cingulate cortex.

    C. Decreased activity in the anterior temporal cortex.

    D. All of the above.

Your answer: ☐

24. A silent cerebral infraction may contribute towards the development of which of the following?

    A. Schizophrenia.

    B. Late-onset depression.

    C. Generalised anxiety disorder.

    D. Increased impulsivity and borderline personality disorder.

Your answer: ☐

25. Seasonal affective disorder demonstrates the influence of which of the following on mood states?

    A. Silent cerebral infraction, dopamine and serotonin.

    B. 5-HT transporters, lipids and the cerebellum.

    C. Lesioning, circadian rhythms and sleep deprivation.

    D. Zeitgebers, circadian rhythms, genetics and 5-HT transporters/receptors.

Your answer: ☐

26. Anticipatory anxiety is consistent with which of the following definitions?

   A. Fear of group participation.

   B. Fear of public speaking.

   C. Fear of having a panic attack.

   D. Fear of contamination.

Your answer: ☐

Extended multiple-choice question

Complete the following caption and diagram using the items listed opposite. Not all of the items will be consistent with the model and not all items can be used. Each item can only be used once.

Figure 1: A diagram representing Selye's (1955) model of the General Adaption Syndrome.

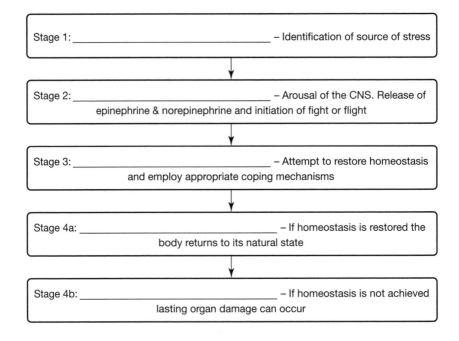

Optional items

A. Alarm reaction

B. Adaption

C. Collapse

D. Exhaustion

E. Inhibition

F. Osmosis

G. Physiological or psychological stressor

H. Resistance

I. Recovery

J. Removal stage

Essay questions for Chapter 6

Once you have completed the MCQs you are ready to tackle the example essay questions below. You might like to select three or four topics and make notes on them. One way of doing this is to create a concept map. The first question has been done for you and you can see how the knowledge required links to some of the MCQs in this chapter.

1. To what extent have biopsychology and other disciplines contributed towards establishing comprehensive and thorough accounts of anxiety and depression?

2. Critically evaluate the methodologies used in biopsychology with reference to the study of emotion.

3. Evaluate the James-Lange theory of emotion with reference to the insights gained from biopsychology.

4. Compare and contrast the evidence provided by neuroimaging and neuropsychology concerning normal and abnormal emotion.

5. To what extent has research with non-human animals contributed towards the contemporary understanding of human emotion?

6. Compare and contrast the evolutionary and cognitive theories of emotion.

7. To what extent are the appraisal, experience and expression of emotion universal phenomena?

8. Critically evaluate the biological approach to studying emotion.

Chapter 6 essay question 1: concept map

To what extent have biopsychology and other disciplines contributed towards establishing comprehensive and thorough accounts of anxiety and depression?

The following concept map presents an example of how your responses to this question could be structured in a meaningful and comprehensive way. There are also links to specific questions in this chapter to guide your revision process. The biological and non-biological factors associated with anxiety, uni-polar depression and bi-polar depression are considered with examples from the chapter.

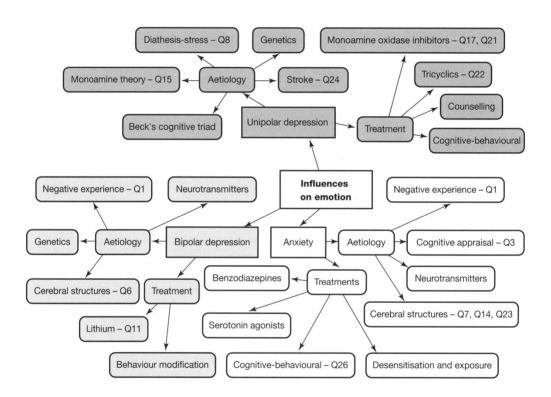

Chapter 7
Learning and memory

This chapter provides questions relating to the biological and psychological factors associated with learning and memory. It includes topics such as schools of thought, key terms and concepts, normal and impaired processing, methodological considerations and prominent milestones in research. It will test both your foundation and advanced knowledge of these topics. At the end of the chapter are several example essay questions and a sample concept map which may enable you to organise your thoughts during essay planning.

Select one answer for each question.

Foundation level questions

1. Which of the following techniques assess implicit memory?

    A. Broken line and mirror drawing.

    B. Free recall and cued recall.

    C. Serial reproduction of text.

    D. Remembering past events and cued recall.

    Your answer: ☐

2. Who stated that if a synapse is repeatedly activated when a postsynaptic neuron fires this will lead to a chemical or structural change which strengthens this connection?

    A. Lashley.

    B. Hebb.

    C. James.

    D. Lange.

    Your answer: ☐

3. Classical conditioning, operant conditioning, reinforcement schedules and motor learning were originally key features in which school of thought?

   A. Cognitive.

   B. Social.

   C. Biological.

   D. Behavioural.

Your answer: ☐

4. Which approach employs experimental and biological techniques to identify normal functioning based on case studies of individuals with impaired functions?

   A. Neuroscience.

   B. Physiology.

   C. Neuropsychology.

   D. Behaviourism.

Your answer: ☐

5. Korsakoff's syndrome presents an example of which of the following conditions?

   A. Retrograde amnesia.

   B. Anterograde amnesia.

   C. Dementia.

   D. Infantile amnesia.

Your answer: ☐

6. Which of the following techniques can be used to assess short-term perceptual memory?

   A. Delayed matching-to-sample task.

   B. Diary keeping.

   C. Serial reproduction.

   D. Word association.

Your answer: ☐

7. The radial maze is designed to test which form of learning?

    A. Declarative memory.

    B. Autobiographical memory.

    C. Semantic memory.

    D. Stimulus–response association.

Your answer: ☐

8. Which of the following terms is consistent with the tendency to report events which did not occur without conscious intention to deceive?

    A. Consolidation.

    B. Confabulation.

    C. Non-declarative.

    D. Construction.

Your answer: ☐

9. By which process may a highly activated synapse lose this strength?

    A. Long-term potentiation.

    B. Short-term potentiation.

    C. Long-term depression.

    D. Short-term depression.

Your answer: ☐

10. Glutamate, dopamine, CaM-KII and NMDA receptors have a significant influence in facilitating which of the following?

    A. Long-term potentiation and learning.

    B. Short-term actualisation and conditioned responses.

    C. Rapid perception and associational learning.

    D. Neurotransmitter transmission and amnesia.

Your answer: ☐

11. Damage to which cerebral area is associated with the inability to perceive and learn visually presented objects?

A. Cerebellum and visual association cortex.

B. Hypothalamus and limbic system.

C. Anterior cingulate cortex and hippocampus.

D. Visual association cortex and inferior temporal cortex.

Your answer:

Advanced level questions

12. By which process is a conditioned response unlearnt?

A. Spontaneous recovery.

B. Extinction.

C. Depolarisation.

D. Potentiation.

Your answer:

13. McDonald and White (1993) observed which of the following effects?

A. Damage to the hippocampal formation only impaired episodic learning.

B. Damage to the amygdala only impaired the ability to learn conditioned associations.

C. Damage to the caudate nucleus and putamen only impaired instrumental learning.

D. All of the above.

Your answer:

14. Damaging or cooling which cerebral structure can impair sensory short-term memory?

    A. Prefrontal cortex.

    B. Left temporal lobe.

    C. Right temporal lobe.

    D. Parietal lobe.

Your answer: ☐

15. Patient WC was able to learn a conditioned emotional response despite damage to which cerebral structure?

    A. Amygdala.

    B. Hypothalamus.

    C. Hippocampus.

    D. Cerebellum.

Your answer: ☐

16. The study of patient HM provided which of the following insights?

    A. Hippocampus does not store or retrieve long-term memories.

    B. Hippocampus does not store immediate short-term memories.

    C. Hippocampus facilitates transition from short- to long-term memory.

    D. All of the above.

Your answer: ☐

17. Patient SM displayed an impaired ability to learn a conditioned emotional response after damage to which cerebral structure?

    A. Amygdala.

    B. Hippocampus.

    C. Hypothalamus.

    D. Prefrontal cortex.

Your answer: ☐

18. Mitsuno et al. (1994) observed that as animals learnt tasks involving the hippocampus they displayed similar changes to those observed during which of the following?

   A. Confabulation.

   B. Long-term potentiation.

   C. Degeneration.

   D. Consolidation.

Your answer: ☐

19. Which cerebral areas are associated with anterograde amnesia?

   A. Limbic cortex, hippocampus and medial temporal lobe.

   B. Cerebellum, hypothalamus and amygdala.

   C. Anterior temporal lobe and prefrontal cortex.

   D. Hippocampus and brain stem.

Your answer: ☐

20. Sullivan et al. (1999) identified that shrinkage of which of the following structures was positively correlated with anterograde amnesia in alcoholics?

   A. Peripheral nervous system synapses.

   B. Cranial nerves.

   C. Mammillary bodies.

   D. White blood cells.

Your answer: ☐

21. Semantic dementia arises due to degeneration of which of the following regions?

   A. Anterior temporal lobes.

   B. Neocortex of lateral temporal lobes.

   C. Prefrontal cortex.

   D. Limbic system.

Your answer: ☐

22. Maguire et al. (2000) observed that London taxi drivers demonstrated which of the following cerebral differences to control subjects after learning locations?

A. Larger posterior hippocampus but smaller anterior hippocampus.

B. Larger ventricle and lateral hippocampus.

C. Smaller posterior hippocampus but larger anterior hippocampus.

D. There were no differences evident using magnetic resonance imaging.

Your answer: ☐

Extended multiple-choice question

Complete the following paragraph using the items listed below. Not all of the items will be consistent with the paragraph and not all items can be used.

Patient HM demonstrated pronounced anterograde amnesia and mild retrograde amnesia for events occurring in the previous two years after a _____ to reduce the effects of convulsions. HM demonstrated that he was unable to learn a series of eight digits even after 25 trials, demonstrating deficits in short-term memory using the _____. Performance on the _____ memory span test also demonstrated that HM was unable to learn the sequence of objects touched by the experimenter, indicating that his amnesia was not restricted to verbal stimuli. However, HM did demonstrate some residual learning on the mirror-drawing task and _____. This suggests that aspects of his _____ remained relatively intact while his declarative knowledge was impaired.

Optional items

A. anterograde

B. cued recall

C. digit-span +1 test

D. block-tapping

E. implicit memory

F. medial temporal lobectomy

G. retrograde

H. rotary-pursuit task

I. semantic memory

J. stroke

Essay questions for Chapter 7

Once you have completed the MCQs you are ready to tackle the example essay questions below. You might like to select three or four topics and make notes on them. One way of doing this is to create a concept map. The first question has been done for you and you can see how the knowledge required links to some of the MCQs in this chapter.

1. Compare and contrast anterograde and retrograde amnesia.

2. To what extent have neuroscience and neuropsychology contributed towards the contemporary understanding of memory?

3. Critically evaluate the strengths and limitations of studying memory from a purely biological perspective.

4. Critically evaluate Hebb's (1949) theory of learning with reference to evidence derived from biopsychology.

5. Compare and contrast the anatomical and physiological factors associated with declarative and non-declarative memory.

6. To what extent can research with non-human animals contribute towards the understanding of human memory?

7. Critically discuss the claim that biological psychology and cognitive psychology provide complementary rather than opposing insights into memory and learning.

8. To what extent can the cerebral structures, physiology and cognitive processes of human memory be said to be universal?

Chapter 7 essay question 1: concept map

Compare and contrast anterograde and retrograde amnesia.

The following concept map presents an example of how your responses to this question could be structured in a meaningful and comprehensive way. There are also links to specific questions in this chapter to guide your revision process. The origins and nature of anterograde and retrograde amnesia are compared and contrasted drawing on examples from the chapter.

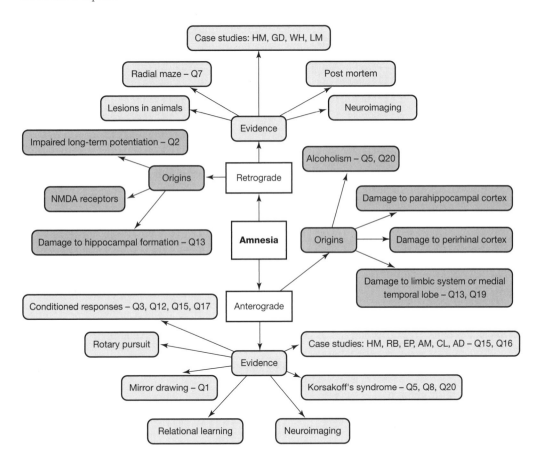

Chapter 8
Language

This chapter provides questions relating to the biological and psychological factors associated with language. It includes topics such as schools of thought, key terms and concepts, normal and impaired processes, methodological considerations and prominent milestones in research. It will test both your foundation and advanced knowledge of these topics. At the end of the chapter are several example essay questions and a sample concept map which may enable you to organise your thoughts during essay planning.

Select one answer for each question.

Foundation level questions

1. The abbreviation LAD in psycholinguistics refers to which of the following hypothetical constructs?

   A. Linguistic-acquisition delay.

   B. Language-acquisition device.

   C. Language-acquisition density.

   D. Language-atrophy device.

   Your answer:

2. In which cerebral area is Broca's area located?

   A. Left hemisphere.

   B. Right hemisphere.

   C. Frontal cortex.

   D. Auditory association cortex.

   Your answer:

3. In which cerebral structure is Wernicke's area located?

   A. Auditory association cortex.

   B. Frontal cortex.

   C. Left hemisphere.

   D. Right hemisphere.

   Your answer: ☐

4. Knecht et al. (2000) observed which pattern of left-hemisphere speech dominance?

   A. 80% of left-handed people, 20% of right-handed people and 90% of ambidextrous people.

   B. 27% of left-handed people, 4% of right-handed people and 15% of ambidextrous people.

   C. 4% of left-handed people, 20% of right-handed people and 3% of ambidextrous people.

   D. 20% of left-handed people, 20% of right-handed people and 25% of ambidextrous people.

   Your answer: ☐

5. Damage to Broca's area is associated with impairment to which of the following?

   A. Language comprehension.

   B. Writing.

   C. Facial discrimination.

   D. Speech production.

   Your answer: ☐

6. Damage to Wernicke's area is associated with impairment to which of the following abilities?

   A. Language comprehension and meaningful speech.

   B. Grammatical production.

   C. Interpretation of non-verbal language.

   D. Writing.

Your answer: ☐

7. Agrammatism is consistent with which of the following definitions?

   A. Difficulty understanding words but comprehension of sentences.

   B. The production of meaningless utterances in Broca's aphasia.

   C. Difficulty understanding and producing grammatical devices.

   D. The lateralisation of language translated to grammatical representations.

Your answer: ☐

8. The KE family experienced a genetic mutation to chromosome seven which led to abnormal development of which cerebral structures?

   A. Wernicke's area and Broca's area.

   B. Caudate nucleus and left inferior frontal lobe.

   C. Right temporal lobe and hippocampus.

   D. Prefrontal cortex and right temporal lobe.

Your answer: ☐

9. Pure word deafness is characterised by which pattern of impairment?

   A. Ability to hear, speak, read and write but not comprehend the meaning of speech.

   B. Ability to comprehend the meaning of speech despite not being able to see text.

   C. Ability to hear and comprehend spoken speech but not text.

   D. Ability to read and hear speech but not produce language.

Your answer: ☐

10. Which of these linguistic tools can be used to convey meaning in speech?

   A. Prosody.

   B. Tone.

   C. Non-verbal gestures.

   D. All of the above.

Your answer: ☐

Advanced level questions

11. Orthographic dysgraphia is a disorder of which form of communication?

   A. Speech production.

   B. Speech perception.

   C. Visually based writing.

   D. Syllabic processing.

Your answer: ☐

12. Activation of the N400 event-related potential indicates which of the following forms of processing?

   A. Semantic processing.

   B. Lexical processing.

   C. Phonological processing.

   D. Perceptual processing.

Your answer: ☐

13. Activation of the P600 event-related potential indicates which of the following violations?

   A. Violations in semantics.

   B. Violations in syntax.

   C. Violations in phonology.

   D. Violations in morphemes.

Your answer: ☐

14. Pure word deafness is produced by which of the following?

   A. Broca's area and occipital cortex.

   B. Cerebellum and left temporal lobe.

   C. Wernicke's area or primary auditory cortex.

   D. Broca's area and right temporal lobe.

Your answer: ☐

15. Damage to which structure has been associated with conduction aphasia?

   A. Lateral Broca's area.

   B. Arcuate fasciculus connecting Wernicke's area and Broca's area.

   C. Anterior Wernicke's area and basal Broca's area.

   D. Parietal cortex and hippocampus.

Your answer: ☐

16. Circumlocutions are often employed by individuals suffering from which condition?

   A. Anomic aphasia.

   B. Secondary anoxia.

   C. Dyslexia.

   D. Dyspraxia.

Your answer: ☐

17. Iacoboni et al. (1999) observed that which cerebral structure was activated when participants observed or copied finger gestures?

   A. Wernicke's area.

   B. Hippocampus.

   C. Broca's area.

   D. Amygdala.

Your answer: ☐

18. Prosody is a function of which cerebral structure also associated with emotional processing and musical skill?

   A. Right temporal lobe.

   B. Left temporal lobe.

   C. Amygdala.

   D. Cingulate anterior gyrus.

   Your answer: ☐

19. Pure alexia is characterised by which pattern of impairment?

   A. Impaired ability to write but unimpaired ability to read.

   B. Impaired ability to speak but unimpaired comprehension.

   C. Impaired speech and comprehension but unimpaired reading.

   D. Impaired ability to read but unimpaired ability to write.

   Your answer: ☐

20. Word-form dyslexia is characterised by which of the following?

   A. Ability to read word but inability to write it.

   B. Comprehension of entire word but not phonemes.

   C. Ability to read a word but only after individual letters are spelled out.

   D. Ability to write complete word but incomprehension of word when spoken.

   Your answer: ☐

Extended multiple-choice question

Complete the areas associated with language on the following diagram using the items listed below.

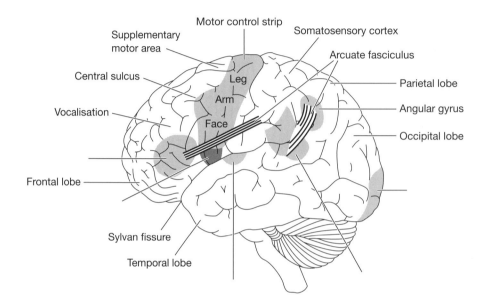

Optional items

A. Brain stem

B. Broca's area

C. Cingulate gyrus

D. Lashley's area

E. Left parietal lobe

F. Primary auditory cortex of motor area

G. Right occipital cortex

H. Visual cortex

I. Vocalisation region of motor area

J. Wernicke's area

Essay questions for Chapter 8

Once you have completed the MCQs you are ready to tackle the example essay questions below. You might like to select three or four topics and make notes on them. One way of doing this is to create a concept map. The first question has been done for you and you can see how the knowledge required links to some of the MCQs in this chapter.

1. Compare and contrast the origins, nature and treatment of Broca's and Wernicke's aphasias.

2. Review the extent to which case studies have contributed towards understanding human language.

3. Compare and contrast the theories, techniques and evidence provided by biopsychology and alternative areas of psychology in regard to language acquisition, production and comprehension.

4. To what extent are language and communication purely human characteristics?

5. Critically evaluate the insights into human language and communication provided by neuroimaging with reference to Broca's and Wernicke's areas.

6. Critically evaluate the theory that speech is primarily a left-hemisphere specialism.

7. To what extent has biopsychology contributed towards understanding language disorders? Discuss with reference to theoretical perspectives, methodologies and research findings.

8. Critically discuss the claim that the bilingual brain contains no differences in structure or processing than the monolingual brain.

Chapter 8 essay question 1: concept map

Compare and contrast the origins, nature and treatment of Broca's and Wernicke's aphasias.

The following concept map presents an example of how your responses to this question could be structured in a meaningful and comprehensive way. There are also links to specific questions in this chapter to guide your revision process. The origins, nature and treatment of Broca's and Wernicke's aphasias are compared and contrasted drawing on examples from the chapter.

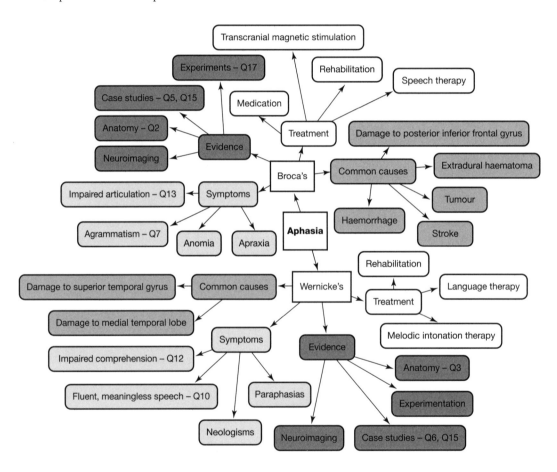

Chapter 9
Consciousness

This chapter provides questions relating to the biological and psychological factors associated with consciousness. It includes topics such as schools of thought, key terms and concepts, normal and altered states, methodological considerations and prominent milestones in research. It will test both your foundation and advanced knowledge of these topics. At the end of the chapter are several example essay questions and a sample concept map which may enable you to organise your thoughts during essay planning.

Select one answer for each question.

Foundation level questions

1. René Descartes advocated which of the following theories?

    A. Monism.

    B. Functionalism.

    C. Dualism.

    D. Structuralism.

    Your answer:

2. Which of the following is not counter-intuitive to Descartes' dualism?

    A. For every conscious experience there is corresponding cerebral activity.

    B. Mind does not exist in the physical dimension.

    C. Drugs alter the state of conscious experience.

    D. Brain damage alters the state of conscious experience.

    Your answer:

3. In Freudian theory, which of the following only operates at an unconscious level?

   A. Ego.

   B. Superego.

   C. Id.

   D. Ego-ideal.

Your answer: ☐

4. Which of the following can alter states of consciousness?

   A. Circadian rhythms.

   B. Substance abuse.

   C. Hypnosis and meditation.

   D. All of the above.

Your answer: ☐

5. Gray's (1971) identity theory is based on which of the following principles?

   A. Mind and brain language discuss the same reality.

   B. Mind and brain language discuss alternate realities.

   C. Mind exists on the spiritual plane while the brain exists on the physical plane.

   D. Brain and mind language discuss alternate states of being.

Your answer: ☐

6. Which of the following changes would result in a shift from automatic functioning to conscious effort?

   A. This would not occur, no processes are actually automatic.

   B. An unexpected change in events or circumstance.

   C. During hypnosis.

   D. When performing a familiar task which requires practised motor movements.

Your answer: ☐

7. MacKay (1987) observed which of the following findings?

   A. Removal of the cerebellum destroys consciousness.

   B. Damage to the limbic system destroys consciousness.

   C. Removal of a cerebral hemisphere does not destroy consciousness.

   D. Removal of the hippocampus does not destroy consciousness.

Your answer:

8. Blindsight is the term assigned to which of the following?

   A. The inability to consciously process unfamiliar objects.

   B. The ability of blind individuals to comprehend objects' functions.

   C. Adaptation of other senses to negotiate blindness.

   D. The ability to reach for an object without conscious experience of it.

Your answer:

9. Hallucinations are prevalent in which of the following conditions?

   A. Schizophrenia and post-traumatic stress disorder.

   B. Chronic depression and bipolar depression.

   C. Generalised anxiety disorder and specific phobia.

   D. Borderline personality disorder and narcolepsy.

Your answer:

10. In which type of study did Sperry (1967) attempt to demonstrate split consciousness?

   A. Cohort study.

   B. Blindsight investigation.

   C. Split-brain study.

   D. Twin study.

Your answer:

11. Which of the following is an accurate description of Baar's (1997) distinction between attention and consciousness respectively?

  A. Both reflect selecting an experience and being aware of this selection.

  B. Selecting an experience versus being aware of selecting an experience.

  C. Both reflect being aware of the selection of experience.

  D. None of the above.

Your answer: ☐

Advanced level questions

12. Wittgenstein (1958) identified which difficulty in testing consciousness and assessing the validity of reports?

  A. Methodologies were technologically insufficient.

  B. Consciousness is private, subjective and cannot be seen by another.

  C. There is not a clear and coherent theory guiding experimentation.

  D. The majority of research had been conducted with non-human animals.

Your answer: ☐

13. Differences in conscious recollection are demonstrated between which of the following?

  A. Declarative and episodic memory.

  B. Language and focused attention.

  C. Implicit and explicit memory.

  D. Perception and language.

Your answer: ☐

14. Kelly (1963) and Rogers (1967) both argued that conscious experience can reveal which of the following?

A. Personality.

B. Intelligence.

C. Unconscious impulses.

D. Psychopathology.

Your answer: ☐

15. Which of the following is observed in cases of anosagnosia?

A. Perception without vision.

B. Drug-induced altered states of consciousness.

C. Inability to consciously identify deficits.

D. None of the above.

Your answer: ☐

16. Split-brain patients are unable to verbally report objects presented to which hemisphere?

A. Right.

B. Both.

C. Neither.

D. Left.

Your answer: ☐

17. Which of the following contains an item not used in medicine to distinguish levels of consciousness?

A. Catatonia and unawareness.

B. Drowsiness and confusion.

C. Normal wakefulness.

D. Coma and semi-coma.

Your answer: ☐

18. Damage to which cerebral structure produces the phenomenon of unilateral neglect?

    A. Occipital lobe.

    B. Right parietal lobe.

    C. Motor cortex.

    D. Left temporal lobe.

    Your answer: ☐

19. Madsen et al. (1991) observed which differences in cerebral activity during REM sleep?

    A. Increase in all areas of the brain.

    B. Decrease in all areas of the brain except the inferior frontal cortex.

    C. Decrease in the occipital cortex but increase in the prefrontal cortex.

    D. Increase in visual association cortex but decrease in inferior frontal cortex.

    Your answer: ☐

20. Which of the following substances is not likely to produce an altered state of consciousness?

    A. MOA inhibitor.

    B. Cocaine.

    C. LSD.

    D. Cannabis.

    Your answer: ☐

21. Scotoma is consistent with which of the following definitions?

    A. Damage to the cerebellum resulting in a lack of consciousness.

    B. Impaired somatosensory system.

    C. Damage to the primary visual cortex resulting in an area of blindness.

    D. Damage to the temporal lobes resulting in split reality.

    Your answer: ☐

22. Patient CK presented an example of which condition?

    A. Apraxia.

    B. Prosopagnosia.

    C. Anoxia.

    D. None of the above.

Your answer: ☐

Extended multiple-choice question

Match the following definitions with the levels of consciousness listed overleaf. Not all of the items will be consistent with the paragraph and not all items can be used. Items can only be used once.

1. The individual can respond to their name and is able to provide information about themselves in a meaningful and appropriate manner. ☐

2. The individual is demonstrating excessive drowsiness and is only able to respond to stimuli in a vague and incoherent manner. ☐

3. The individual demonstrates little interest in or awareness of their surroundings and any responses are slow. ☐

4. The individual is not consciously aware but will react to unpleasant stimuli with withdrawal and expression. ☐

5. The individual shows vital signs but does not present any discernable consciousness, cannot be woken and does not respond to stimuli. ☐

(For optional items see overleaf)

Optional items

A. Abnormal

B. Chemical

C. Comatose

D. Declined

E. Normal wakefulness

F. Obtunded

G. Redundant

H. Regressive

I. Somnolent

J. Stuporous

Essay questions for Chapter 9

Once you have completed the MCQs you are ready to tackle the example essay questions below. You might like to select three or four topics and make notes on them. One way of doing this is to create a concept map. The first question has been done for you and you can see how the knowledge required links to some of the MCQs in this chapter.

1. To what extent can biopsychology investigate consciousness? Discuss with reference to a minimum of two topics (e.g. drug abuse and brain damage).

2. Critically evaluate the claim that consciousness cannot be studied or measured but rather exists on a spiritual plane.

3. To what extent does substance abuse alter the state and function of consciousness?

4. Discuss and review the study of consciousness in contemporary psychology with specific reference to neuropsychology and neuroimaging.

5. Critically discuss the extent to which the study of consciousness has been facilitated by technological and theoretical advancements.

6. Compare and contrast monist and dualist perspectives on consciousness with reference to the methodologies employed in biopsychology and experimental findings.

7. Critically discuss and evaluate the theory that meditation and hypnosis can significantly alter the state of consciousness without the use of medication, cortical stimulation or lesions.

8. To what extent can neuroimaging and neuropsychology contribute towards the understanding of consciousness?

Chapter 9 essay question 1: concept map

To what extent can biopsychology investigate consciousness? Discuss with reference to a minimum of two topics (e.g. drug abuse and brain damage).

The following concept map presents an example of how your responses to this question could be structured in a meaningful and comprehensive way. There are also links to specific questions in this chapter to guide your revision process. The various areas of study, methodologies, strengths and limitations relating to studying consciousness are incorporated into the concept map drawing on examples from the chapter.

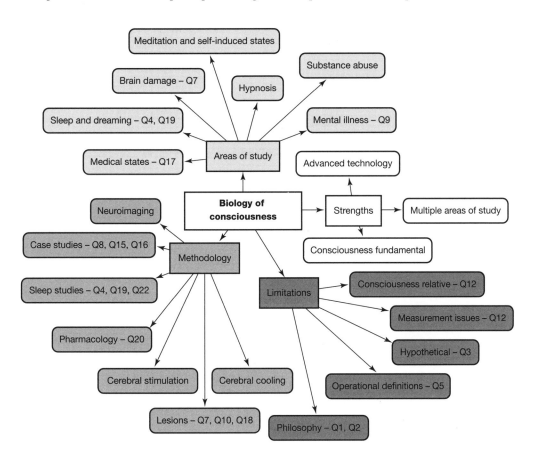

Chapter 10
Behavioural genetics

This chapter provides questions relating to the field of behavioural genetics. It includes topics such as schools of thought, key terms and concepts, individual differences, clinical psychology, methodological considerations and prominent milestones in research. It will test both your foundation and advanced knowledge of these topics. At the end of the chapter are several example essay questions and a sample concept map which may enable you to organise your thoughts during essay planning.

Select one answer for each question.

Foundation level questions

1. Which of the following techniques is often used in behavioural genetics?

    A. Twin studies.

    B. Adoption studies.

    C. Family studies.

    D. All of the above.

    Your answer: ☐

2. Heredity is consistent with which of the following definitions?

    A. The extent to which a behaviour or characteristic is due to genetics or the environment.

    B. The extent to which a behaviour aids survival of the fittest.

    C. The extent to which mutation has altered the genetic chain.

    D. The extent to which a characteristic is changeable within a community.

    Your answer: ☐

3. Which of the following groups share the greatest proportion of their genetics?

    A. Dizygotic twins.

    B. Monozygotic twins.

    C. Fathers and sons.

    D. Siblings.

Your answer: ☐

4. Epigenetics is the study of which behavioural change?

    A. How DNA continually changes throughout the lifespan.

    B. How genetic mutation upon conception alters the traits of the offspring.

    C. How the environment contributes to behaviour irrespective of genetics.

    D. How the environment causes genetic traits to be expressed differently.

Your answer: ☐

5. Natural selection is consistent with which of the following definitions?

    A. Inherited traits which provide selective advantages prevail.

    B. Genetic mutation facilitates diversity in the gene pool but may not be advantageous.

    C. All traits and types serve a specific function even if maladaptive.

    D. Mate selection is the product of pheromones and likelihood of successful reproduction.

Your answer: ☐

6. Which of the following are believed to have a genetic component?

    A. Schizophrenia and depression.

    B. Intelligence and personality.

    C. Skills and anxiety disorders.

    D. All of the above.

Your answer: ☐

7. Which of the following cannot confound measures of personality?

    A. Leading or double-barrelled questions.

    B. Social desirability and demand characteristics.

    C. Measurement error and poor standardisation.

    D. None of the above.

Your answer: ☐

8. Which of the following is not a test of reliability on an intelligence or personality measure?

    A. Test-retest.

    B. Alternate forms.

    C. Predictive test.

    D. Split half.

Your answer: ☐

9. What did Mischel (1968) argue influenced personality?

    A. Genetics.

    B. Situations.

    C. Physiology.

    D. Cerebral activity.

Your answer: ☐

10. Which of the following tests do not assess intelligence?

    A. Factor Five.

    B. Wechsler's.

    C. Stanford-Binet.

    D. Raven's.

Your answer: ☐

11. Which of the following points can confound evidence concerning the nature–nurture debate?

   A. Genetics can determine the nature of the environment individuals seek.

   B. A specific cause of a behaviour rarely occurs in isolation.

   C. Humans are complex organisms which cannot be studied in a vacuum.

   D. All of the above.

   Your answer: ☐

12. The condition phenylketonuria (PKU) arises due to the mutation of how many genes?

   A. Four.

   B. Three.

   C. One.

   D. Two.

   Your answer: ☐

Advanced level questions

13. Loehlin (1992) reviewed which two forms of study in an attempt to identify the heredity of Costa and McCrae's (1992) five personality traits?

   A. Twin and adoption.

   B. Family and population.

   C. Screening and family.

   D. Questionnaires and experiments.

   Your answer: ☐

14. Lynn (2001) agued for which of the following principles?

   A. Social constructionism.

   B. Eugenics.

   C. Genetic engineering.

   D. None of the above.

   Your answer: ☐

15. Tyron (1940) selectively bred which of the following?

    A. Aggressive and passive monkeys.

    B. Rats differing in temperament.

    C. Maze bright and maze dull rats.

    D. Monkeys differing in intelligence.

Your answer: ☐

16. Kangas and Bradway (1971) observed which correlation between general intelligence measures taken in childhood and adulthood?

    A. 0.80.

    B. 0.67.

    C. 0.52.

    D. 0.41.

Your answer: ☐

17. Bouchard and McGue (1981) attributed what proportion of variance in IQ to genetics?

    A. 50%.

    B. 80%.

    C. 20%.

    D. 15%.

Your answer: ☐

18. Plomin (1988) identified which correlations in IQ scores for identical twins reared together and apart respectively?

    A. 0.87 and 0.74.

    B. 0.50 and 0.82.

    C. 0.69 and 0.62.

    D. 0.91 and 0.23.

Your answer: ☐

19. Rose (1988) identified which correlations in neuroticism scores for identical and fraternal twins respectively?

A. 0.69 and 0.70.

B. 0.38 and 0.15.

C. 0.41 and 0.22.

D. 0.81 and 0.66.

Your answer: ☐

20. Gametes are processed by which of the following processes?

A. Mitosis.

B. Meiosis.

C. Diffusion.

D. Alleles.

Your answer: ☐

21. Gottesman and Bertelsen (1989) observed that which percentage of schizophrenic and non-schizophrenic monozygotic twins carried the 'schizophrenia gene'?

A. 17.4% and 2.1%.

B. 5.8% and 18.3%.

C. 23.6% and 20.2%.

D. 16.8% and 17.4%.

Your answer: ☐

22. Rosenthal (1971) identified that individuals with a close relative with an affective disorder are how much more likely to experience the condition than those without afflicted relatives?

A. 20 times more likely.

B. 5 times more likely.

C. 10 times more likely.

D. 30 times more likely.

Your answer: ☐

23. On which chromosome(s) is a 'bipolar gene' believed to potentially reside?

   A. 4, 5, 18, 21 of X.

   B. All chromosomes.

   C. 2, 8, 9, 10, 11, 13, 22 of Y.

   D. 11, 13, 14, 15, 19 of X.

Your answer: ▢

24. Which of the following terms refers to traits which occur in one of two forms?

   A. Monozygotic traits.

   B. Dichotomous traits.

   C. Dizygotic traits.

   D. Heterozygous traits.

Your answer: ▢

Extended multiple-choice question

Complete the following paragraph using the items listed opposite. Not all of the items will be consistent with the paragraph and not all items can be used.

Several methodologies have been developed to study the influence of genetics and the environment on traits and behaviours. This ratio is often referred to as _____ and reflects the proportion of variance on any given trait which may be explained by the environment and genetics respectively. For example, twin studies investigate the degree of similarity shared between siblings. This technique relies on the assumption that _____ will demonstrate the greatest degree of similarity due to sharing an identical genetic chain. However, _____ can also be used to investigate the variance explained by both genetic and _____ factors. However, this involves several ethical issues including a potential invasion of privacy. Another approach which has been highly criticised for ethical reasons is the use of _____. Researchers using this approach genetically engineer mutated genes in a laboratory and observe the effects when these are introduced into the chromosomes of mice.

Optional items

A. adoption studies

B. dizygotic twins

C. environmental

D. fraternal twins

E. heredity

F. inheritance

G. monozygotic twins

H. magnetic resonance testing

I. targeted mutations

Essay questions for Chapter 10

Once you have completed the MCQs you are ready to tackle the example essay questions below. You might like to select three or four topics and make notes on them. One way of doing this is to create a concept map. The first question has been done for you and you can see how the knowledge required links to some of the MCQs in this chapter.

1. To what extent has behavioural genetics clarified the traits and behaviours which are acquired through heredity?

2. Critically discuss the nature–nurture debate with reference to intelligence and mental health.

3. Critically evaluate the extent to which personality is a product of the environment and upbringing rather than genetics.

4. To what extent has research demonstrated that developmental and mood affective disorders are hereditary?

5. Critically evaluate the argument that schizophrenia is an inevitable disorder in families with a history of the condition.

6. To what extent have the methods of behavioural genetics contributed towards the contemporary understanding of individual differences and heredity?

7. Critically discuss the validity and reliability of measures in behavioural genetics with reference to both genetic screening and experimental approaches.

8. To what extent do the findings derived from behavioural genetics support the theory of evolution? Discuss with reference to both healthy and maladaptive behaviours.

Chapter 10 essay question 1: concept map

To what extent has behavioural genetics clarified the traits and behaviours which are acquired through heredity?

The following concept map presents an example of how your responses to this question could be structured in a meaningful and comprehensive way. There are also links to specific questions in this chapter to guide your revision process. The various influences of genetics and the environment are considered and evaluated with reference to methodologies, areas of study and issues and debates.

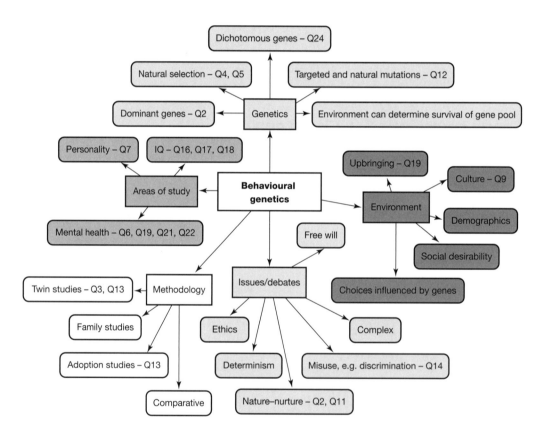

Writing an essay: a format for success

The following bullet points provide you with some general guidance for essay writing and are intended to assist you in formulating and arranging your arguments. However, remember that the structure may vary according to topic and the nature of the essay question. For further guidance concerning the American Psychological Association's style please consult the APA guidelines.

- All essays should begin with a brief introduction summarising the scope and direction of your response to the question and the conclusions which will be drawn. You should assume that the reader of your essay will have no previous knowledge of the subject and so write as clearly and explicitly as possible.

- It is recommended that you establish your stance early in the essay to provide a strong foundation for debate and consideration of evidence.

- The next section of your essay should briefly present the theories which will be critically evaluated throughout the essay. All technical terms should be clearly defined to demonstrate knowledge and make the essay accessible to the reader. The original sources for the theories and any relevant adaptations should be cited fully in the APA format.

- All of the relevant aspects of the theories should be discussed, evaluated and, ideally, compared. For example, does one of the theories present a more comprehensive account than the alternative perspectives or do the theories review the same phenomenon at complementary but alternative levels of analysis? The student should also make explicit references to how an analysis of each theory would facilitate a response to the question.

- You must also be careful to establish a balance between descriptive and critical writing. For example, essays which compare and contrast perspectives and evidence will achieve better results than those which only reiterate information with no analysis.

- Research evidence supporting and refuting each theory should be presented and critically reviewed. This evidence should be synthesised rather than simply restated. For example does the majority of evidence support one theory or are there remaining flaws with the account? All sources must be cited fully and should be drawn from appropriate material.

- Always link each paragraph back to the essay question to explain how the text has answered the question and to maintain a clear progression in your argument.

- Base your conclusion on the weight of the evidence supporting each argument. The conclusion should be written clearly with direct links back to the essay question. While the consideration of the evidence should be balanced, this does not prevent you from adopting a perspective.

- All sources used throughout the essay should be cited in APA format in a reference list if the essay is submitted as an assignment. If the essay is submitted in examination conditions, the guidelines for your particular institution should be consulted.

Scoring methods in MCQs

Introduction

All assessments need to be reviewed and marked. At your university you will come across a number of formal (often called summative) and informal (aka formative) assessments. These can take the form of practical reports, essays, short-answer questions and (of course) examinations. There are, of course, a number of forms of examinations – short answers, written essays and multiple-choice questions (or MCQs).

MCQs are considered objective assessments, that is answers are unambiguously correct or incorrect and therefore provide for high marker reliability – so that's one positive mark for MCQs. On the other hand, there is often a concern (for the examination setter) that guessing by the candidate can have an inflationary influence on the marks. By chance, if you have four choices then you should score 25% just by guessing. This is obviously not a situation to be encouraged, and because of this your psychology course team may have introduced various attempts to make sure that this does not happen. It is worth exploring some of these methods and the implications these will have for the approach you take to your assessment and, ultimately, how they can impact on your examination performance.

Scoring of MCQ examinations can take several forms. At its most simple, a raw score is calculated based on the total number of correct responses (usually 1 mark per correct answer). Under this approach, any omissions or incorrect responses earn you no marks but neither do they attract a penalty. If you get the question right, you get a mark; if you do not then you get no mark.

As mentioned, alternative and more complex approaches to marking have been developed because of concerns that results can be inflated if correct responses are the result of successful guessing. The most common approaches to discouraging random guessing include the reward of partial knowledge and negative marking. This can impact on your behaviour and your learning. Of course, whatever the examination and whatever the marking scheme, you need to know your stuff!

Rewarding partial knowledge

Scoring procedures developed to reward partial knowledge are based on the assumption that though you and your student colleagues may be unable to identify a single correct response you can confidently identify some options as being incorrect and that partial knowledge should therefore be rewarded. Versions of this approach generally allow you to choose:

- more than one possibly correct response and to be awarded a partial mark provided one of your responses is the correct answer;
- a 'not sure' option for which you are awarded a proportion of a mark (usually either 0.2 or 0.25).

Negative marking

Negative marking is when your performance is based on the total number of correct responses which is then reduced in some way to correct for any potential guessing. The simplest application of negative marking is where equal numbers of marks are added or subtracted for right and wrong answers and omitted answers, or the selection of a 'No answer' option that has no impact on marks. So, you get +1 mark when you get the question right, −1 mark when you get it wrong and 0 if you do not attempt it. However, there are other approaches which are slightly more punitive. In these approaches, if you get the question correct you get +1, if you get the question wrong then this is awarded a −1 (or even −2) and if there is no attempt then this is awarded a −1 as well as, it is suggested, you do not know the answer.

How does this impact on you?

The impact of these scoring mechanisms can be significant. By way of example, use the following table to demonstrate your performance in each of the chapters in this text. For each of the chapters work out the number of correct responses (and code this as NC), the number of incorrect answers (coded as NI) and the number of questions that you did not provide a response to (NR). You can then use the formulae in the table to work out how you would have performed under each of the different marking schemes. For example, for the punitive negative marking scheme you score 18 correct (NC=18), 2 incorrect (NI=2) and omitted 5 questions (NR=5). On the basis of the formula in the table, NC-(NI*2)-NR, you would have scored 9 (i.e. 18-(2*2)-5). So even though you managed to get 18 out of 25 this would have been reduced to only 9 because of the punitive marking.

Chapter	Number correct	Number incorrect	No response	Marking scheme: raw score	Marking scheme: partial knowledge	Marking scheme: negative marking	Marking scheme: punitive negative marking
	NC	NI	NR	= NC	= NC – (NI * 0.2)	= NC – NI	= NC – (NI * 2) – NR
1							
2							
3							
4							
5							
6							
7							
8							
9							
10							
TOTAL							

Explore the scores above – which chapter did you excel at and for which chapter do you need to do some work? Use the above table to see your areas of strength and areas of weakness – and consequently where you need to spend more time revising and reviewing the material.

MCQ answers

Chapter 1: Introduction to biological psychology – MCQ answers

Level	Question number	Correct response	Self-monitoring
Foundation	1	D	
Foundation	2	A	
Foundation	3	B	
Foundation	4	C	
Foundation	5	A	
Foundation	6	B	
Foundation	7	D	
Foundation	8	A	
Foundation	9	B	
Foundation	10	C	
Foundation	11	A	
Foundation	12	D	
Advanced	13	B	
Advanced	14	A	
Advanced	15	C	
Advanced	16	D	
Advanced	17	A	
Advanced	18	B	
Advanced	19	A	
Advanced	20	D	
Advanced	21	C	
Advanced	22	B	
Advanced	23	A	
Advanced	24	C	
Advanced	25	B	
Advanced	26	B	
		Total number of points:	Foundation: Advanced:

EMCQ for Chapter 1

The correct responses are provided below. A maximum of 5 points can be allocated.

1. An approach which studies the neurological basis of behaviour and experience. = **E**

2. An approach which attempts to identify the cerebral structures associated with normal functioning by studying individuals with impaired functioning. = **I**

3. An approach which attempts to investigate and manipulate neural activity using various medications. = **F**

4. An approach which attempts to identify the correlates between physiology and psychological processes. = **G**

5. An approach which employs techniques such as fMRI to study the neural basis of cognition. = **A**

Chapter 2: The nervous system – MCQ answers

Level	Question number	Correct response	Self-monitoring
Foundation	1	D	
Foundation	2	A	
Foundation	3	B	
Foundation	4	C	
Foundation	5	A	
Foundation	6	D	
Foundation	7	A	
Foundation	8	C	
Foundation	9	B	
Foundation	10	A	
Foundation	11	A	
Foundation	12	D	
Advanced	13	B	
Advanced	14	C	
Advanced	15	D	
Advanced	16	A	
Advanced	17	B	
Advanced	18	C	
Advanced	19	D	
Advanced	20	A	
Advanced	21	B	
Advanced	22	A	
Advanced	23	D	
		Total number of points:	Foundation: Advanced:

EMCQ for Chapter 2

The paragraph should read as follows. A maximum of 5 points can be allocated.

The human nervous system is a complex organisation consisting of several branches and complex neural pathways. For example, the <u>central nervous system (CNS)</u> incorporates the brain and spinal cord and is responsible for several regulatory processes and cognition. In contrast, the <u>peripheral nervous system (PNS)</u> consists of all of the nerves and ganglia located beyond the central nervous system. This system functions primarily as a connection to the central nervous system although some of the pathways, such as the <u>enteric nervous system</u>, can function independently. The PNS can also be differentiated by two prominent overarching systems. The <u>somatic nervous system</u> consists of efferent nerves and is responsible for controlling voluntary movement. In contrast the <u>autonomic nervous system</u> consists of both afferent and efferent neurons and primarily operates beyond consciousness.

Chapter 3: Sensory systems I – MCQ answers

Level	Question number	Correct response	Self-monitoring
Foundation	1	A	
Foundation	2	B	
Foundation	3	D	
Foundation	4	A	
Foundation	5	C	
Foundation	6	B	
Foundation	7	A	
Foundation	8	D	
Foundation	9	D	
Foundation	10	C	
Foundation	11	A	
Foundation	12	B	
Advanced	13	A	
Advanced	14	D	
Advanced	15	B	
Advanced	16	A	
Advanced	17	C	
Advanced	18	A	
Advanced	19	A	
Advanced	20	B	
Advanced	21	C	
Advanced	22	A	
Advanced	23	D	
Advanced	24	B	
		Total number of points:	Foundation: Advanced:

EMCQ for Chapter 3

The paragraph should read as follows. A maximum of 5 points can be allocated.

The somatosensory system is a complex and diverse aspect of the human organism which monitors and responds to information obtained from <u>bodily senses</u>. Indeed, Pinel's (2003) model of the system incorporates hierarchical, cascading and parallel processing between the central nervous system and <u>peripheral nervous system</u>. For example, the <u>association cortex</u> transmits information to the secondary motor cortex, primary motor cortex, brain stem motor nuclei and spinal motor circuits. However, transmission of information also occurs within and between these other structures via <u>descending motor circuits</u>. Furthermore, information is transmitted from muscles and the peripheral nervous system to each level of the central nervous system via <u>feedback circuits</u>. This demonstrates the complex and vital nature of this system.

Chapter 4: Sensory systems II – MCQ answers

Level	Question number	Correct response	Self-monitoring
Foundation	1	A	
Foundation	2	C	
Foundation	3	B	
Foundation	4	D	
Foundation	5	A	
Foundation	6	B	
Foundation	7	A	
Foundation	8	D	
Foundation	9	B	
Foundation	10	C	
Foundation	11	A	
Advanced	12	D	
Advanced	13	C	
Advanced	14	A	
Advanced	15	B	
Advanced	16	A	
Advanced	17	B	
Advanced	18	D	
Advanced	19	A	
Advanced	20	C	
Advanced	21	B	
Advanced	22	D	
		Total number of points:	Foundation: Advanced:

EMCQ for Chapter 4

The correct responses are provided below. A maximum of 5 points can be allocated.

1. This term is assigned to the system consisting of semicircular canals and receptor organs in the inner ear. = **J**

2. This term is assigned to the sensory system which is responsible for taste. = **B**

3. This term is assigned to the sensory system which is responsible for smell. = **E**

4. This term is assigned to the dendrites of mitral cells and the terminal buttons of axons in the sensory system responsible for smell. = **F**

5. This term is applied to the taste sensation produced by glutamate. = **I**

Chapter 5: Motivation – MCQ answers

Level	Question number	Correct response	Self-monitoring
Foundation	1	D	
Foundation	2	C	
Foundation	3	B	
Foundation	4	D	
Foundation	5	A	
Foundation	6	B	
Foundation	7	C	
Foundation	8	A	
Foundation	9	B	
Foundation	10	D	
Foundation	11	A	
Advanced	12	C	
Advanced	13	A	
Advanced	14	C	
Advanced	15	A	
Advanced	16	D	
Advanced	17	B	
Advanced	18	A	
Advanced	19	D	
Advanced	20	A	
Advanced	21	B	
Advanced	22	A	
Advanced	23	C	
		Total number of points:	Foundation: Advanced:

EMCQ for Chapter 5

The correct responses are provided below. A maximum of 5 points can be allocated.

1. A condition characterised by excessive body mass index which places the individual at risk of health problems, specifically heart disease and stroke. = **I**

2. A condition characterised by sporadic binging and purging which can harm the digestive tract. = **D**

3. A condition characterised by under-consumption, serious health complications and an emaciated appearance. = **B**

4. A condition characterised by the uncontrollable, sporadic need to sleep. Also often categorised by cataplexy, sleep paralysis and hypnagogic hallucinations. = **H**

5. A condition characterised by an inability to sleep despite an often strong motivation to do so. = **F**

Chapter 6: Emotion – MCQ answers

Level	Question number	Correct response	Self-monitoring
Foundation	1	D	
Foundation	2	B	
Foundation	3	C	
Foundation	4	D	
Foundation	5	A	
Foundation	6	B	
Foundation	7	D	
Foundation	8	C	
Foundation	9	A	
Foundation	10	B	
Foundation	11	D	
Foundation	12	A	
Foundation	13	C	
Advanced	14	A	
Advanced	15	B	
Advanced	16	C	
Advanced	17	B	
Advanced	18	D	
Advanced	19	A	
Advanced	20	A	
Advanced	21	C	
Advanced	22	D	
Advanced	23	D	
Advanced	24	B	
Advanced	25	D	
Advanced	26	C	
		Total number of points:	Foundation: Advanced:

EMCQ for Chapter 6

The diagram should look as follows. A maximum of 5 points can be allocated.

Figure 1: A diagram representing Selye's (1955) model of the General Adaption Syndrome.

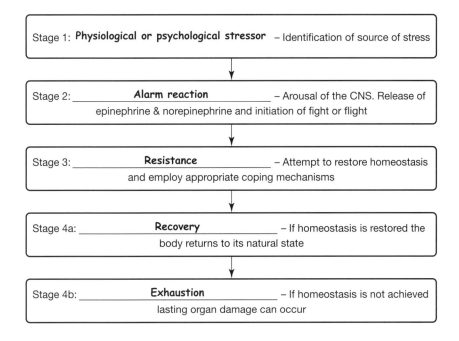

Stage 1: **Physiological or psychological stressor** – Identification of source of stress

Stage 2: _____ **Alarm reaction** _____ – Arousal of the CNS. Release of epinephrine & norepinephrine and initiation of fight or flight

Stage 3: _____ **Resistance** _____ – Attempt to restore homeostasis and employ appropriate coping mechanisms

Stage 4a: _____ **Recovery** _____ – If homeostasis is restored the body returns to its natural state

Stage 4b: _____ **Exhaustion** _____ – If homeostasis is not achieved lasting organ damage can occur

Chapter 7: Learning and memory – MCQ answers

Level	Question number	Correct response	Self-monitoring
Foundation	1	A	
Foundation	2	B	
Foundation	3	D	
Foundation	4	C	
Foundation	5	B	
Foundation	6	A	
Foundation	7	D	
Foundation	8	B	
Foundation	9	C	
Foundation	10	A	
Foundation	11	D	
Advanced	12	B	
Advanced	13	D	
Advanced	14	A	
Advanced	15	C	
Advanced	16	D	
Advanced	17	A	
Advanced	18	B	
Advanced	19	A	
Advanced	20	C	
Advanced	21	B	
Advanced	22	A	
		Total number of points:	Foundation: Advanced:

EMCQ for Chapter 7

The paragraph should read as follows. A maximum of 5 points can be allocated.

Patient HM demonstrated pronounced anterograde amnesia and mild retrograde amnesia for events occurring in the previous two years after a medial temporal lobectomy to reduce the effects of convulsions. HM demonstrated that he was unable to learn a series of eight digits even after 25 trials, demonstrating deficits in short-term memory using the digit-span +1 test. Performance on the block-tapping memory span test also demonstrated that HM was unable to learn the sequence of objects touched by the experimenter, indicating that his amnesia was not restricted to verbal stimuli. However, HM did demonstrate some residual learning on the mirror-drawing task and rotary-pursuit task. This suggests that aspects of his implicit memory remained relatively intact while his declarative knowledge was impaired.

Chapter 8: Language – MCQ answers

Level	Question number	Correct response	Self-monitoring
Foundation	1	B	
Foundation	2	C	
Foundation	3	A	
Foundation	4	B	
Foundation	5	D	
Foundation	6	A	
Foundation	7	C	
Foundation	8	B	
Foundation	9	A	
Foundation	10	D	
Advanced	11	C	
Advanced	12	A	
Advanced	13	B	
Advanced	14	C	
Advanced	15	B	
Advanced	16	A	
Advanced	17	C	
Advanced	18	A	
Advanced	19	D	
Advanced	20	C	
		Total number of points:	Foundation:\nAdvanced:

EMCQ for Chapter 8

The diagram should look as follows. A maximum of 5 points can be allocated.

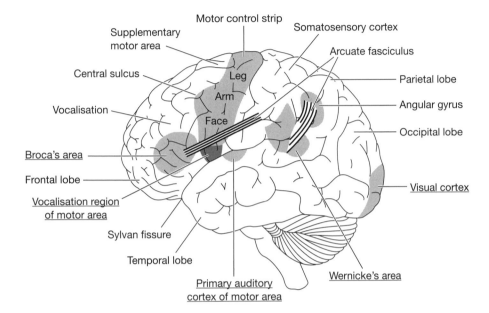

Chapter 9: Consciousness – MCQ answers

Level	Question number	Correct response	Self-monitoring
Foundation	1	C	
Foundation	2	B	
Foundation	3	C	
Foundation	4	D	
Foundation	5	A	
Foundation	6	B	
Foundation	7	C	
Foundation	8	D	
Foundation	9	A	
Foundation	10	C	
Foundation	11	B	
Advanced	12	B	
Advanced	13	C	
Advanced	14	A	
Advanced	15	C	
Advanced	16	D	
Advanced	17	A	
Advanced	18	B	
Advanced	19	D	
Advanced	20	A	
Advanced	21	C	
Advanced	22	B	
		Total number of points:	Foundation: Advanced:

EMCQ for Chapter 9

The correct responses are provided below. A maximum of 5 points can be allocated.

1. The individual can respond to their name and is able to provide information about themselves in a meaningful and appropriate manner. = **E**

2. The individual is demonstrating excessive drowsiness and is only able to respond to stimuli in a vague and incoherent manner. = **I**

3. The individual demonstrates little interest in or awareness of their surroundings and any responses are slow. = **F**

4. The individual is not consciously aware but will react to unpleasant stimuli with withdrawal and expression. = **J**

5. The individual shows vital signs but does not present any discernable consciousness, cannot be woken and does not respond to stimuli. = **C**

Chapter 10: Behavioural genetics – MCQ answers

Level	Question number	Correct response	Self-monitoring
Foundation	1	D	
Foundation	2	A	
Foundation	3	B	
Foundation	4	D	
Foundation	5	A	
Foundation	6	D	
Foundation	7	B	
Foundation	8	C	
Foundation	9	B	
Foundation	10	A	
Foundation	11	D	
Foundation	12	C	
Advanced	13	A	
Advanced	14	B	
Advanced	15	C	
Advanced	16	D	
Advanced	17	A	
Advanced	18	A	
Advanced	19	C	
Advanced	20	B	
Advanced	21	D	
Advanced	22	C	
Advanced	23	A	
Advanced	24	B	
		Total number of points:	Foundation: Advanced:

EMCQ for Chapter 10

The paragraph should read as follows. A maximum of 5 points can be allocated.

Several methodologies have been developed to study the influence of genetics and the environment on traits and behaviours. This ratio is often referred to as <u>heredity</u> and reflects the proportion of variance on any given trait which may be explained by the environment and genetics respectively. For example, twin studies investigate the degree of similarity shared between siblings. This technique relies on the assumption that <u>monozygotic twins</u> will demonstrate the greatest degree of similarity due to sharing an identical genetic chain. However, <u>adoption studies</u> can also be used to investigate the variance explained by both genetic and <u>environmental</u> factors. However, this involves several ethical issues including a potential invasion of privacy. Another approach which has been highly criticised for ethical reasons is the use of <u>targeted mutations</u>. Researchers using this approach genetically engineer mutated genes in a laboratory and observe the effects when these are introduced into the chromosomes of mice.